Ask the Body,
and Treat the Priority

by Molly Jones L.Ac., Dipl. Ac.

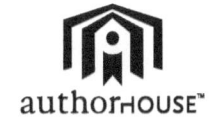

author**HOUSE**™

1663 LIBERTY DRIVE, SUITE 200
BLOOMINGTON, INDIANA 47403
(800) 839-8640
WWW.AUTHORHOUSE.COM

First published by AuthorHouse 05/17/05

ISBN: 1-4208-4545-4 (sc)

Printed in the United States of America
Bloomington, Indiana

This book is printed on acid-free paper.

Cover art and illustrations by Molly Jones

To Chuck, P.K., and Sunny

Acknowledgments

Many thanks to my clients who pushed me to develop the skills mentioned in this book. To Dr. Latifa Amdur who traded many fine vial based treatments with me since 1996. To the doctors of vibrational medicine who developed this revolutionary form of treatment. And to Adi Da Samraj, whose spiritual transmission opened my brain and made me more psychic.

Other books by Molly Jones

The Sky Goes on Forever, written and illustrated by Molly Jones, under the name Molly MacGregor

The Magnificent Trickster: The Story of Milarepa, written and illustrated by Molly MacGregor

Vegetable Surrender, written by Adi Da Samraj, illustrated by Molly MacGregor

White Magic, Vibrational Medicine in Action, written and illustrated by Molly Jones (out of print.)

Table of Contents

Chapter One 1
Treat the Priority

Chapter Two..15
Case Histories

Chapter Three..31
Dowsing with a Pendulum

Chapter Four 35
How I Developed as an Intuitive Healer

Chapter Five..41
White Magic - Vibrational Medicine in Action, Revisited

Chapter Six..45
Treating Fatigue

Chapter Seven 51
Treating the Digestion

Chapter Eight 57
Treating Emotions

Chapter Nine 61
Treating the Brain and Nervous System

Chapter Ten...65
Treating Bacterial and Viral Infections

Chapter Eleven..69
Osteoporosis

Chapter Twelve 77
A Discussion of Diet

Chapter Thirteen 83
Treating Addictions

Chapter Fourteen..85
Treating Children and Animals

Appendix 1 87
Resource

Appendix 2...91
Menus

Bibliography 95

Introduction

This book is about how to treat people more effectively by asking the client's body every step of the way.

The material presented here is written primarily for acupuncturists who know several techniques, including one or more vibrational medicine techniques such as Nambudripad's Allergy Elimination Technique (NAET), Total Body Modification (TBM), Jaffe-Mellor Technique (JMT), Body Alignment Technique (BAT), or Bioset. Chiropractors, naturopaths, and M.D.'s similarly trained can also make use of the information on treating by priority. The book is written in a simple enough style to appeal to a general reader who wishes to know more about optimizing treatment using vibrational medicine.

I am an acupuncturist also trained in several vibrational medicine techniques including NAET, JMT, BAT, and TBM. I also prescribe herbs and other naturopathic remedies, as well as dietary changes when called for. I have tried using various diagnostic machines (like the Voll and Bioset machines) but do not resonate well with these tools, so instead rely on muscle testing and dowsing with a pendulum to ask the body.

I use the technique of asking the body and treating by priority on virtually every client because I prefer this way of treating. You may choose to do this, or you may reserve this skill to work on problem cases that no one else can figure out.

No one practitioner has all the answers or is correct all the time. No one treatment modality is perfect. However, you can treat by asking the body and treating by priority to get better results overall, and you can use the techniques you are already trained in and the tools you already have to do this.

Chapter One
Treat the Priority

The first step in learning how to ask the body is to throw away your theories about how to treat, and any standard protocol that may be lodged in your brain. Each treatment is determined according to each individual's needs by asking their higher intelligence via their body exactly what to do. Keep an open mind at all times.

When I began working in vibrational medicine I noticed that clients were energetically weak on many, many vials. I would stand there muscle testing someone and often find scores of vials they were weak on, *apparently* needing to be cleared on. Also, often they were showing weaknesses on many organs, glands, systems, and specific points when muscle tested.

For example, they might come in showing energetic weakness on the liver, spleen, colon, lungs, and many glands. They could have apparent food intolerance, sensitivities to man made substances such as plastics, pesticides, and herbicides, and indications of the possible presence of many parasites when muscle tested on these individual vials.

People sometimes brought in computer print outs with hundreds of items on them that they were apparently energetically weak on. (The parasite list always makes people feel hysterical.) Often those who sought treatment would look aghast at the long list of items it seemed necessary to test for and clear. Even getting people to come in for ten successive treatments was sometimes difficult.

I struggled with this dilemma for some time and then decided that there had to be a quicker way to work. I have found that working based on *priority* (a concept borrowed from Dr. Jeff Levin, the developer of Body Alignment Technique) works quickly and effectively to sweep away many energetic abnormalities at once.

When the practitioner treats based on the client's priority, the energetic integrity of their body is strengthened at a deep level. In the process, many other energetic weaknesses will be strengthened automatically. It is not necessary to clear vials just because a client shows weakness in response to them. When you treat the priorities many vials strengthen automatically.

The first thing I do when a new client comes in is fill out an intake report. Then the client lies down and I muscle test for any weakness anywhere in the body. I muscle test all over the body to see if there are any weaknesses.

If the client has mentioned an area that is bothering them, I muscle test that area. For example, if someone says their hip is bothering them I muscle test the hip. If someone says their brain function is bothering them I muscle test the brain. Invariably these areas will test weak.

All practitioners who have trained in vibrational medicine have been taught how to muscle test the body to check for abnormalities on organs, glands, systems, and points. Thus, I do not have to teach that information here.

The key to successful treatment is to treat the body so that all areas become normalized and stay normalized from week to week. The client should also test well on most vials you challenge them with. The way to get these results is to *accurately treat by priority.*

I usually muscle test with the arm at a 45 degree angle. Sometimes a client will have a lot of arm strength, so I use an even lesser 30 degree angle. Sometimes a client has very little arm strength so I muscle test with the arm at a 90 degree angle. I find that testing *with the fist* closed gives a more accurate reading. While touching an organ, gland, or point I push down and if the arm gives way, the area I am testing is abnormal.

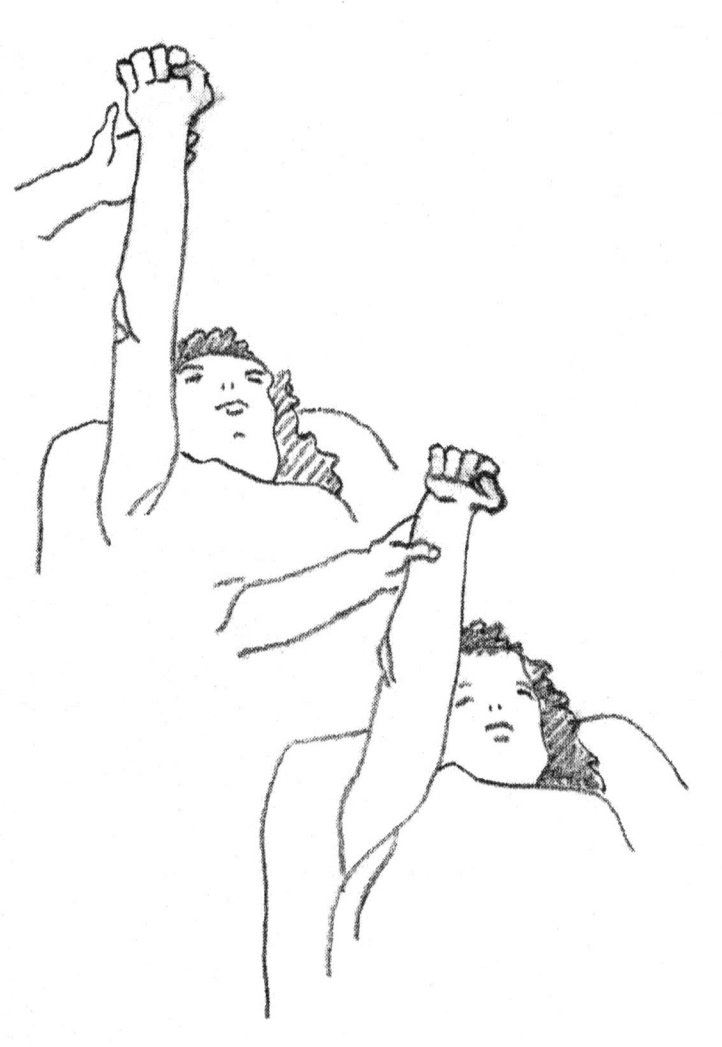

How do you get the client's readings to hold strong from week to week so that they don't need as much treatment? *By treating their priorities.* How do you get many vials to clear automatically? *By clearing their priority vials.* How do you get vials to clear on the first try? *By clearing their priority vials.* It is a dead give away that you are not treating by priority if you have to clear a vial more than once or (rarely) twice.

This is not rocket science, folks. In order for the client to feel better they must have normal, stable readings. They will feel this change if you treat their priorities accurately. Treating by priority is primarily for practitioners working in vial based techniques. However, any practitioner who knows several techniques can treat by priority using the following step by step protocol.

Steps in determining and treating each individual's priorities:

1. Make sure you and client are hydrated.

2. Establish testability.

3. Menu your repertoire of treatment modalities, and determine the first treatment modality used to do the first priority.

4. Ask detailed and specific questions to determine exactly how to treat the first priority, and treat as indicated.

5. Continue the same procedure for the next priority, and so on.

6. Double check readings on organs, glands, systems, and points. Treat local problems if necessary.

7. Work until you get a "hands off" reading.

8. "Lock in" the treatment.

Step 1: Make sure you and client are hydrated.

Most people walk around in a state of partial dehydration. This means that both you and the client need to drink water before a treatment in order to get accurate readings. I often drink two to three eight ounces of water before I start working. I continue drinking frequently during the time I am treating people. Often I drink a liter of water during each 45 minute treatment session. This is especially important in getting accurate readings when dowsing with a pendulum, less important when muscle testing.

Step 2: Establish "testability."

With the client lying on the treatment table, ask the body if there is enough awareness for accurate testing. I call this "testability." The body needs testability in order to answer your questions accurately.

If you do not get a positive response, testability is easily established by treating auricular points Helix #4 and Helix #5. You may use a needles, laser, or magnets to treat these points. (You may also establish testability by using the "awareness" balance in TBM, if you are trained in this modality.) Ask the body how long these points need to be treated for each individual.

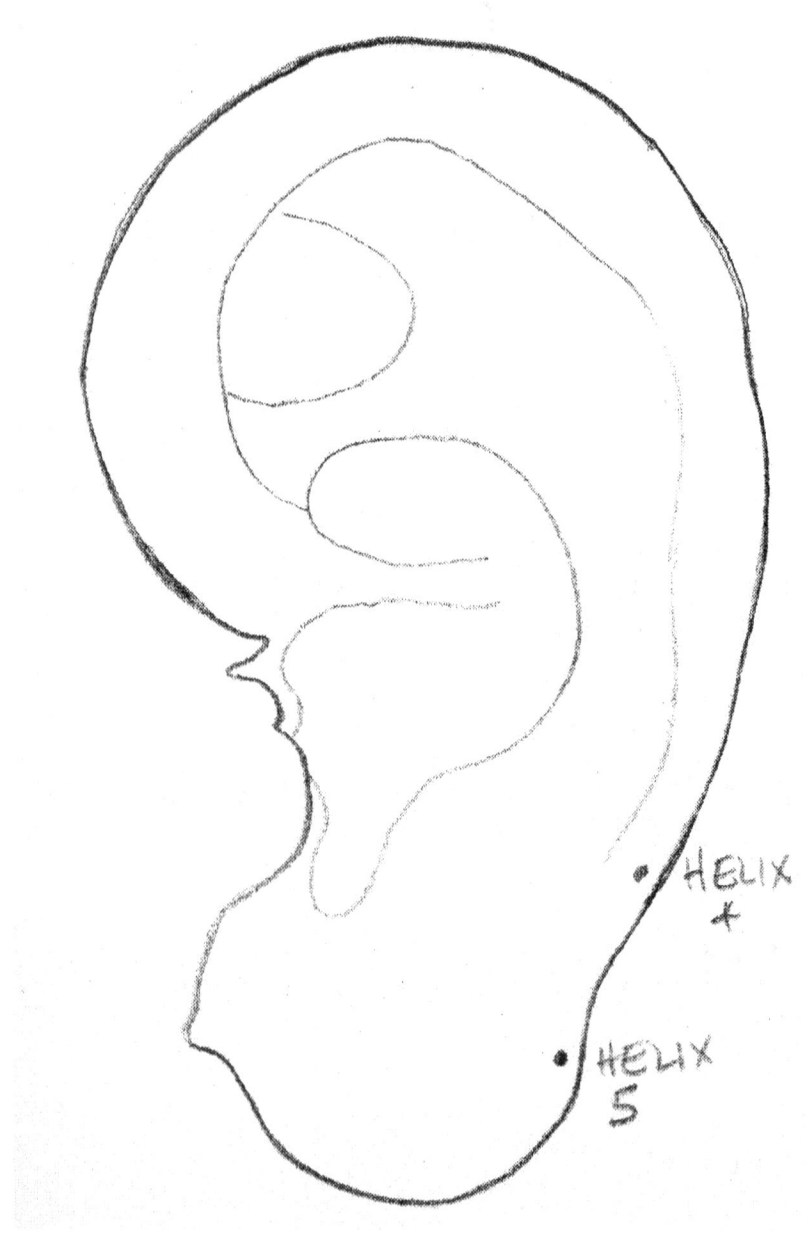

Step 3: Menu your repertoire of treatment options, and determine the first treatment modality used to do the first priority.

The name of this book should actually be "Ask **Higher Intelligence** via the Body and Treat the Priority." *The client's higher intelligence is aware of every procedure you can do and every tool, supplement, herbal formula, and vial you have in your office that you are familiar with.* This intelligence will be able to tell you exactly what to do if you ask the right questions. This intelligence will also take into account the amount of time you have to treat them, treatment modalities you are strongest in, and your skill level.

*Asking the body will work if you ask **specific detailed** questions, while remaining **neutral**.* If you have an agenda and are not asking from a neutral disposition you can throw the readings. Ask "yes" or "no" questions. Speak out loud, while muscle testing after each question. You may also internally verbalize your questions if you one pointedly direct your mental attention toward the body of the client while touching them.

I do not use the protocol of asking questions of the clients left brain rather than the right brain as taught by some teachers, as I find that often the (supposedly) illogical treatment priorities given by a dominant right brain work very well to correct imbalances.

Here are sample questions that I personally use to begin a treatment, based on menuing my entire repertoire of treatment modalities:

"Does this individual need TBM?"

"Treatment using NAET vials?"

"JMT vials?"

"BAT balances?"

"Acupuncture?"

"Another modality?" (see additional modality list in appendix #2)

Molly Jones L.Ac., Dipl. Ac.

I muscle test with each question, and if the arm gives way that indicates a "yes" to me. (I find this type of muscle testing much better because the arm only gives way with a "yes", not with each "no" response. There will be fewer "yes" responses than "no" responses, and thus less strain on the client's arm during testing.)

Step 4: Ask detailed and specific questions to determine exactly how to treat the first priority, and treat as indicated.

The answer to the first series of questions in Step 3 tells me what modality to use to treat their first priority.

For example, if the answer is "acupuncture," I then ask in a series of questions about *exactly* how to do the acupuncture treatment:

"Should I begin working on: the spleen meridian?"

"liver meridian?"

"stomach meridian?"

"gallbladder meridian?" and so on.

Once I get that answer I ask about individual points on that meridian to determine which point or points to use. I usually ask about the distal "command" points first, since those are the ones most commonly used. I then will move to the body points and the auricular points. For example, if the spleen meridian is to be worked on first I ask:

"Should I use spleen 3?"

"spleen 4?"

"spleen 6?" and so on.

I will begin needling, based on the information I have received. I then continue to muscle test, asking for more points using specific questions about which other meridians to use and points within those meridians. I continue needling based on this information, until all needles are placed. At a certain point there will be no more points indicated as necessary by the body.

I then double check and make sure by asking if all needles have hit the points and are understood by the body. This is necessary because often the simplest part of the treatment is overlooked - that all the points are hit! The body will tell you if the points are not understood.

I then ask how long the needles need to be left in (one minute? two minutes? five minutes? ten minutes?, etc.), wait, and then remove as indicated. Occasionally some needles are removed before others. Then I ask the body if there is another priority. Usually there is.

Step 5: Continue the same procedure to determine the next priority, and so on.

Again, I run a series of questions by muscle testing:

"Do you need TBM?"

"Treatment using NAET vials?"

"JMT vials?"

"BAT balances?"

"More acupuncture (now an unlikely option.)?"

"Another modality?"

Perhaps the body indicates a JMT vial. I have three JMT boxes of vials and I ask:

"Is the vial in box 1?"

"box 2?"

"box 3?"

After getting that answer I go through the columns in the correct box until I get the correct column. Then I ask:

"Is the vial in the top third of the column?"

"The middle third?"

"The bottom third?"

That answer narrows down field of vials more, until I can hone in on the correct vial. I place the vial on the thymus and ask the body if this is the correct vial:

"Is this the correct vial?"

Their arm must give way when you muscle test, otherwise it is not the right vial. If the body indicates it is the correct vial, I then ask if there any other adjunct vial or vials that need to be placed on the thymus with the priority vial. Sometimes there are, sometimes not. If there are, I repeat the procedure to find the correct adjunct vial or vials. It could be any vial in your office!

Once I find the priority vial and any adjunct vial or vials I then ask specific questions by muscle testing on *exactly* how to clear the vial. There are techniques within each system to clear vials, so I ask:

"Should I use the JMT clearing protocol?

"The NAET clearing protocol?"

"TBM clearing protocol?"

"Specific unusual acupuncture points to clear the vial?" (These are often auricular points.)

Once I get this information I clear the priority vial and adjunct vials if there are any, *using the clearing technique required for this individual for this particular vial.*

Once this priority is completed, I ask if there is another priority and continue the treatment in the same manner. Usually there are three or four priorities per treatment, but there may be more on certain clients. If there is a *particular* vial I wish to clear I ask the body's permission. If I get an okay, I will go ahead and clear it. I always double check to see if there are any preparatory priorities necessary to complete before clearing the vial. This preparatory work ensures that the vial will clear on the first try and will also minimize treatment reactions. If you do not get permission to clear a vial in any particular session, *don't clear it*! The body is not ready, but may be at some future time after more priority work is done.

Step 6: Work until you get a "hands off" reading.

I work until there are no more priorities indicated by the body that day, except for local problems. I do not treat beyond this point. By treating accurate priorities and honoring the body's "hands off" answer you will absolutely minimize treatment reactions. Any time you have to repeatedly clear a vial you *know* it is not a priority vial.

I do not subscribe to the belief that getting worse after a treatment is a sign of a healing crisis. Nine times out of ten getting worse is an indicator of an incorrect treatment by the practitioner. Clients should enjoy more ease, greater stability of health, and decreased symptoms if treatments are correct. The exception to this is a detoxification problem that arises after a correct treatment. The body may get backed up and need help in detoxifying. Again, the body itself will tell you if this is the case and what organ or organs need help detoxifying.

Molly Jones L.Ac., Dipl. Ac.

Step 7: Double check all readings on organs, glands, systems and points.

I go back and double check everything, especially a problem area that the client mentioned earlier. If you accurately treat the priorities the readings should be strong.

The priorities should directly relate to the client's root level imbalances. For example, I treated a lady with cerebral palsy whose brain readings were weak. Her priorities were neurotransmitter and heavy metals balances. After treating these priorities the readings on her brain came up, indicating that the priorities were accurate.

Sometimes the priorities will make logical sense to you, and sometimes not. Don't worry about it! When you treat priorities accurately the readings *will* normalize, whether or not the priorities make logical sense.

There may still be a weak reading on a local problem, which is more superficial. If this is the case, I ask the body for permission to treat this local problem, particularly if it is an area that is bothering the client. Clients with long term chronic health problems may not give permission to treat a local problem after treating their priorities, because it is too much for their system to handle. If I get permission I treat the local area, using the modality most appropriate as indicated by the body. I always check the reading after treating a local problem. It should be holding strong.

For example, someone may have had knee surgery and still need local acupuncture needles around the knee after their major priorities are treated. I often send people home with small Korean hand magnets to place on the area to keep the readings strong during the week.

Some people come in *just* for local treatment. They are not interested in deeper level work and want symptomatic relief for a local problem. If this is the case I skip the deeper level priority treatments and use standard acupuncture treatment and/or herbs. I treat them for a relatively short period of time this way, at the most six treatments. If they get enough relief, great! If not, I try to lean them toward getting prioritized treatments at this point, since their superficial problem may be deeper than we originally thought.

On clients with long term chronic health problems there may be some readings that don't come up after you have completed treating them for the day. Since you have a "hands off" indication you are finished for that day in any case. You *will* achieve more rapid, deeper results and greater stability on all readings when you treat accurately by priority.

People should not wait forever to get results. I expect to see results in three or four treatments with most people, and within three months on people with severe chronic illness.

Step 8: Lock in the treatment.

After completing a treatment that has included vibrational work "lock in" the information by blocking the client with chiropractic blocks. Ask the body if "locking in" is necessary, as sometimes it is not.

If so, the high hip gets a block between the twelfth rib and the apex of the hip, while the low hip gets a block at the gluteal crease. Ask the body which is the high hip. Ask the body how long the blocks are retained for each individual.

TBM and BAT have more complex "locking in" procedures, and if you know these procedures you may choose to use one of them. In general, however, blocking is sufficient.

Chapter Two
Case Histories

All treatments are determined individually by asking the body, step by step in detail.

#1 Single 49 year old male with left sided pain including the toes, knee, hip, and shoulder. He reports feeling "way out of balance." He mentions being sexually abused as a child. He is a carpenter. There is heavy toxin exposure in this profession, although he has been using a respirator and gloves in recent years. He is also receiving chiropractic treatments which he likes. In checking the body, the whole left side is weak.

1. Establish testability. This is done before each treatment by asking the body if there is enough "awareness" for testing to be accurate.

2. TBM is the first modality:
TBM balance of head of pancreas
TBM balance of invasion syndrome (see below re: TBM module 1)

3. First priority vial is 'nitrate/nitrite' vial, cleared using TBM clearing protocol. (All vials are placed on the thymus to clear.)

4. Next priority is a TBM 'emotional' vial using TBM clearing protocol.

5. Next priority vial is another TBM 'emotional' vial using TBM clearing protocol.

6. Next priority is acupuncture: pericardium 7, triple heater 6, liver 3, right auricular point for heart.

7. Hands off, lock in. Left side readings are normal, all readings normal.

Please note: *TBM practitioners are asked to clear the entire first module before proceeding. However, after establishing testability I have found that you can effectively treat by priority.*

In this particular case history, treating the head of pancreas and doing the "invasion" balance as the first priority brought up the rest of the module 1 readings automatically.

TBM practitioners can verify the effectiveness of treating by priority for themselves. *Establish "awareness", then check everything in the first module without correcting anything. Treat the priorities one by one until the treatment is complete. Go back and double check your module 1 readings. If you have accurately treated the priorities you will find that most and, often all module 1 weaknesses have strengthened automatically.*

TBM practitioners can also follow the standard TBM protocol of bringing up everything in the first module before going on to the client's priorities.

Client returns two weeks later, feels "much better." Left side reading is normal, now the right side is weak. Testability is already established.

1. First priority is acupuncture: gallbladder 37, liver 5 (both junction pts.) bilateral.

2. Second priority is a TBM 'emotional' vial cleared using TBM protocol.

3. Third priority is acupuncture: spleen 4, stomach 40 (both junction pts.) bilateral.

4. Hands off, lock in. All readings both left and right are normal.

Client returns two months later. All readings are normal at the start of the treatment. He has fallen in love with a high school sweetheart. He would like to be cleared for smoking. Testability is already established.

1. First priority is TBM invasion syndrome balance.

2. Permission to clear TBM 'smoking' vials is given by the body. These vials were cleared using spinal cord auricular point on the back of the right ear.

I could have used standard acupuncture treatment on this client. Why work by priority using more modalities? Because you can work at a deeper level. Readings will normalize faster and there will be greater stability.

#2 59 year old woman with multiple symptoms including headaches, achy joints, fatigue, muscle aches, gas and bloating, and a compromised immune system. In 1976 she had ovarian cancer and had a complete hysterectomy. She reports receiving NAET treatments for several years including the standard protocol of clearing the basics, as well as clearing herpes, shingles, mononucleosis, EBV, coxsackie virus, and meningitis.

Her practitioner had done a good job on this difficult case. However, results were still limited. She still has multiple symptoms and is not well. Her stability is compromised on a daily basis. Testability is established.

1. The first priority is 'tumor' vial plus 'herpes simplex II' as the adjunct vial. These vials were cleared using a BAT balance for residue, plus the heart point in the right ear.

17

2. 2nd priority is real 'blood' (pin-prick to get a drop of real blood) plus actual 'black' color, cleared using the first part of the BAT sensitivity balance. (This priority is straight from the right brain! There is no theoretical left brained logic that could explain this one.) Hands off, lock in.

The client returns the within the next few days "feeling better." Testability is established.

1. 'Blood' plus 'black' color cleared using the second part of the BAT sensitivity balance.

2. 'Stealth pathogen' vial cleared using a BAT sensitivity balance. Hands off, lock in.

The client returns home, on another island. She reports feeling better and greater stability in many ways over the next several weeks.

How do you unlock a difficult case such as this one? By treating by priority. How do you work on a client that has had extensive vibrational medicine work already, with limited results? By accurately treating the priorities.

#3 The client is a 47 year old woman who reported problem with fatigue and her digestion. She stated that both kidneys were bothering her and that she had pain in the jaw behind the teeth on the left side. All symptoms started after she had a dental procedure involving injection of a medication. She feels she reacted to the injection.

1. Testability was already established. TBM liver balance, balance for both kidneys, and free radicals balance. (Anytime a free radical balance is done I always check to see if the client needs to go on an oral antioxidant, which in this case she did.)

2. Acupuncture points on the liver meridian: liver 3 and 8 bilateral.

Also colon 4, and auricular point for the mouth, left side only.

3. Clear a vial for 'injected toxins' plus adjunct 'blood' vial cleared using TBM protocol. I asked permission to clear this vial. Hands off, lock in.

She returned in one week reporting all symptoms better, but not completely gone. She reported smelling strange smells such as alcohol, and burning hair. This information came out after I gave her time to talk while I rummaged around in my desk. I used this unusual signal from the body to determine the next priorities. Testability is already established.

1. Acupuncture: gallbladder 41 and triple heater 5, extraordinary meridian points needled bilaterally. (If the body indicates a master point, I will automatically ask if the coupled point should be used with it. In this case the answer was "yes".)

2. The body indicated another modality - detoxification - was needed. After some detective work this seemed to be scrubbing the skin on the face for ten minutes a day for three days. This was a skin detox measure near the injection site.

3. Cleared 'human hair' vial using the auricular mandible pt. left side.

4. Cleared 'bourbon' vial using the auricular maxilla pt. left side, plus heart 9 on the left. Hands off, lock in.

She returned one week later saying everything was "much better."

1. Acupuncture: small intestine 19 on the left side only with a magnet.

Molly Jones L.Ac., Dipl. Ac.

2. Cleared a vial for 'synergistic toxins' cleared using auricular mouth point left side. I asked permission to clear this vial after determining it was her priority vial.

3. Stomach 12 with a magnet, left side only. Hands off, lock in.

She reported that all symptoms resolved after this treatment. All readings were normal after the third treatment. The reading on the left side of the jaw at the injection site was the last one to come up.

#4 20 year old female college student who was "sick a lot during the first part of the school year" and had since been experiencing multiple food allergies. She reports particular problems with gluten. *She is weak on the gluten vial as well as **all** of the basics.* She already has testability.

1. First priority is a TBM (unusual) 'virus' vial plus 'blood' X 2. I used both TBM blood vials here, although it could be done with two separate drops of actual blood on cotton balls. I always ask if real blood needs to be used or not. If real blood is required the client can lance their own finger if necessary. Cleared using TBM protocol. Hands off, lock in.

She came back one week later.

1. Priority was TBM long allergy procedure using the TBM three vial protocol. This protocol clears many food allergies in one fell swoop. There is no avoidance period. Hands off, lock in.

She came back two weeks later, not holding the last treatment. ***This is a dead give away that there is something else going on.***

1. I could not get permission to do any modality that I do in my practice. So I went to the modalities list (see appendix 2) and found she needed cranio-sacral work. Luckily this young woman's parents are both massage therapists and could do cranio-sacral work themselves. This was done within the next two days. *She came back*

after two days and the TBM long allergy procedure treatment was now holding. I did not repeat this treatment. Also, five of the basics had come up automatically.

1. The next priority was 'gluten' plus 'blood' X 3 cleared using the NAET clearing protocol. I used two TBM blood vials plus one drop of actual blood on cotton to get blood X 3, all placed on the thymus. Hands off, lock in. *After this treatment gluten and all but two of the basics had cleared. These vials cleared automatically.*

    Case #4 is a good case history for NAET practitioners to see the effectiveness of treating by priority. *In this case priority treatments strengthened the basics automatically. Also, in this case some of the priorities had to do with food allergies, but I have seen the basics come up automatically without treating **any** food allergy priority.* ***Simply treat the priorities as you find them!***
    The fact that a treatment was "lost" showed immediately that there was something else prior that needed to be done so that the treatment would hold, in this case cranio- sacral work.
    *Please note: NAET practitioners should complete work on the basics before moving on to treat by priority **if** they have formally agreed to follow standard NAET protocol.*

#5 This client is a 42 year old man with pain in his sacrum on the left side. His general initial reading is weak everywhere, including the left sacrum. Testability was already established. Here I worked by priority to establish greater stability throughout the whole body, then worked on the local area.

1. First priority is acupuncture: conception vessel 24. (*No* other points were indicated as necessary by the body!) This brings up all readings except the left sacrum.

2. The second priority is 'blood waste' vial cleared using the auricular upper back point (back of the right ear.) Hands off, lock in.

3. Local treatment of acupuncture on the sacrum points: bladder 31, 32, 33 bilateral. I also placed one magnet on the governor vessel line at gv 2. These points brought up the reading on the sacrum area. The client was given magnets to place on the painful spots of the sacrum as necessary while he slept. He called back in a week and said the sacrum pain was gone.

#6 56 year old woman with a lingering viral or bacterial infection. She has gone to a conventional M.D. and an M.D. specializing in complementary treatment but is still healing very slowly. She has a cough and is fatigued.

1. Testability is already established. First priority is TBM module 3 respiratory balance.

2. 'Blood waste' vial plus actual 'blood' cleared using auricular spinal cord point on the back of the ear.

3. Acupuncture: liver 13, 14, colon 4, lung 1

4. 'Richettsia' vial cleared using TBM protocol. Hands off, lock in.

   She returns a week later feeling better, but still with a sense that the infection is lingering within her system in some way. Testability is established.

1. TBM digestive system balance

2. Acupuncture: stomach 42, small intestine 3, plus auricular small intestine point.

3. 'Virus mix' vial cleared using auricular spinal cord point on the back of the ear.

4. Modality: increase live food (raw) by 30%.

5. 'Infectious mononucleosis' vial cleared using the auricular "stop wheezing" point on the right ear. Hands off, lock in.

She returns in one week, feeling much better. Testability is established.

1. TBM crop protection vials cleared using TBM protocol.

2. Acupuncture: triple heater 23 right side only, gallbladder 41 with triple heater 5 (extra meridian points) needled bilaterally. After asking the body I used ion pumping cords on these four points. Hands off, lock in.

#7 A young female college student comes in complaining of pain whenever she eats, no matter what she eats. After eating she craves sugar. When I ask her if she has gas and bloating she says "yes!" She has been to a conventional allopathic doctor with no result. I check the root cause list (see appendix 2) and dowse the information "candida." She reports that she had the NAET basics done earlier in the year, but none of them are holding at this time. Testability is already established.

1. The first priority is acupuncture: spleen 4 with pericardium 6 using ion pumping cords.

2. Correct sex II, a TBM balance.

3. Clear 'staphylococcus' vial using TBM protocol. (She then reports that she has had a staph infection during the first semester.)

4. Acupuncture: spleen 6

5. Clear five vials at once: 'candida', 'mold', 'blood' X 2, and 'alcohol', using TBM protocol. All are placed on the thymus. Hands off, lock in. She was put on a candida diet consisting of animal protein and non starchy vegetables plus olive leaf extract.

Molly Jones L.Ac., Dipl. Ac.

She returns the next day reporting "almost no stomach pain." Testability is established.

1. Acupuncture: small intestine 3.

2. Clear a TBM 'emotional vial' using TBM protocol.

3. Acupuncture: liver 3.

4.TBM three vial allergy protocol using the long procedure. After completing this treatment the basics are holding *automatically.*

5. *Very hidden (*See how to find hidden priorities in chapter 6) reading: 'herpes simplex' vial cleared using the colon point, both ears. Hands off, lock in.

She returns the next day reporting "stomach even better." Testability is established.

1. TBM 'crop protection' vials cleared with TBM protocol.

2. Cleared 'hormone mix' vial plus 'blood' X 3 using TBM protocol.

3. Acupuncture: small intestine 3. Hands off, lock in.

The following day she returns for the final treatment before returning to college. She will maintain the candida diet for about a month and continue taking olive leaf extract during that time. If the diet is constipating she is to take more fiber in the form of psillium and/or more vegetables. After a month she can slowly incorporate more unrefined carbohydrates. Testability is already established.

1. BAT motion balance to correct trauma from a recent automobile accident.

2. Acupuncture: small intestine 7.

3. Clear 'live vaccine' vial plus 'blood' X 2 using TBM protocol.

4. Clear vial for 'menstrual flow' using TBM protocol. Hands off, lock in.

#8 67 year old woman who had her right upper lung removed two years ago because of a cancerous tumor. She is in remission. She is somewhat short of breath upon exertion, and is using a steroid inhaler. She has recently had NAET treatments to clear the basics as well as a few other vials. The basics are holding.

In checking the root cause for cancer I find the answer "inflammation in the lungs." (This information was quickly determined by dowsing the root cause list, followed by dowsing a menu for organs, glands, and systems in different parts of the body.) In questioning the body as to whether there is still inflammation the answer is "yes." Further questioning of the body as to the cause of inflammation yields the answer "infection in the venous system of the lungs." She lives elsewhere, so treatments are concentrated within a short period of time.

1. Establish testability.

2. Acupuncture: colon 11, small intestine 7.

3. Clear vial for 'synergistic poisons' using TBM protocol.

4. Clear 'printing mix' vial using auricular lateral lung points.

5. Real 'blood' plus 'tumor' vial cleared using middle back point back side of right ear.

5. Hands off, lock in.

Second treatment, the next day:

Molly Jones L.Ac., Dipl. Ac.

1. Testability is already established. Acupuncture: kidney 22 - 27 bilateral.

2. BAT meridian balance.

3. 'Medications mix' vial cleared using full JMT protocol.

4. Modality needed: cranio-sacral work, particularly addressing the occipital bones. She will get this work done when she returns home. This modality request was repeated several times by the body, indicating the importance of having cranio-sacral work done. Hands off, lock in.

    Third treatment, the next day:

1. Testability is already established. Acupuncture: kidney 10 bilateral.

2. BAT balance for circulation access point combined with 'iG mix' vial.

3. Cleared her steroid inhaler using full NAET protocol.

4. Cleared scar weakness from surgery using directional eye movement technique for scars. Hands off, lock in.

    Fourth treatment, the next day:

1. Testability is already established. 'Streptococcus' vial (very hidden weakness on this vial) cleared using a laser on the inside and outside of the ears, plus needling the auricular lateral lung point on the right side.

2. 'Blood' X 4 cleared using TBM 'T cell' vials protocol. Because the body indicated real blood was necessary, I used four drops of real blood on separate balls of cotton placed on the thymus. Hands off, lock in.

After the fourth treatment the reading on inflammation in the lungs was finally better, and the reading on an infection in the venous system was better as well.

Fifth treatment, the next day:

1. Testability is already established. TBM 'crop protection' vials plus adjunct 'blood' vial cleared using TBM protocol.

2. 'Adrenal' vial plus 'corticosterone' vial plus adjunct 'blood' vial cleared by using TBM protocol. Hands off, lock in.

The client returned home where she will get cranio-sacral work as indicated as important by the body. I will check her through her hair (which acts as an energetic witness) via distance to be sure that the inflammation readings and infection readings stay normal. This is extremely important in this case to help insure no reoccurrence of cancer. In checking for inflammation and infection each area of the lung is checked in *minute* detail using a diagram of the lungs because a general overall reading is not sufficient in this case.

#9 A 45 year old woman with erratic periods, lots of hot flashes and night sweats.

First treatment:

1. Establish testability.

2. TBM pancreas balance.

3. TBM hepatic system balance.

4. Clear 'hormone' vial with TBM protocol.

Molly Jones L.Ac., Dipl. Ac.

5. Acupuncture: gallbladder 41 with triple heater 5, bilateral with ion pumping cords.

6. Three Immortals herbal formula for menopausal symptoms. Hands off, lock in.

Second treatment:

1. Testability is established. Acupuncture: spleen 6; small intestine 3 with bladder 62, bilateral with ion pumping cords.

2. BAT meridian balance.

3. Kidney 6 with lung 7, bilateral with ion pumping cords. Hands off, lock in.

Third treatment:

1. Establish testability.

2. 'Medications mix' vial cleared using TBM protocol.

3. Acupuncture: spleen 6.

4. TBM endocrine system balance.

5. Acupuncture: triple heater 5 with gallbladder 41, bilateral with ion pumping cords crossing from left to right and visa versa. Hands off, lock in.

Fourth treatment:

1. Establish testability.

2. Acupuncture: bladder 60.

3. 'Insulin' vial cleared using auricular adrenal points. Hands off, lock in.

Fifth treatment:

1. Testability is established. 'Epinephrin' vial cleared using spinal cord #2 point on the back of the right ear.

2. TBM adrenals balance with 'iG mix' vial cleared using TBM protocol and spinal cord #1 auricular point on the back of the left ear. Hands off, lock in.

Client reports one hot flash per week at this point.

1. Establish testability.

2. Acupuncture: small intestine 3 with bladder 62, bilateral with ion pumping cords.

3. Clear (a different) 'hormone mix' vial using TBM protocol. Hands off, lock in.

#10 Client is a forty year old woman with multiple complaints including "no functioning immune system," and "brain problems." She has a history of lung infections, chronic fatigue, cognition problems, and repeated colds and flues. She is currently receiving blood injections for the immune system from a naturopathic physician. She is also receiving treatment from another naturopathic practitioner. Testability is already established.

I do not receive any information on priorities to do on this client. None of my standard modalities are usable, nor are any other modalities. I then dowse the BAT emotions menu which has hundreds of words related to emotional conditions. I receive the information "hopeless" and "hypochondriac." This client is then gently directed to look at her root level mental mistake of seeing herself as a sick person. She is also given a booklet on right thinking written by the late William W. Walter, a metaphysical practitioner. His teaching clearly explains the relation of right thinking to health, and sick thinking to disease. No other treatment is indicated as necessary at this time.

Most people that I treat are willing to actively, persistently visualize themselves as being healthy along with treatment. In this case, this practice was this client's number one priority.

Chapter Three
Dowsing with a Pendulum

I prefer dowsing with a pendulum over muscle testing. It is faster and takes less work because you don't have to put repeated downward pressure on the client's arm while asking the body.

It is also easier to get incorrect readings when using a pendulum, a real drawback when you are asking the body. The success of your treatments depends on getting accurate readings! When I first started using a pendulum I always double checked my readings with muscle testing, and I *still* do this fairly regularly.

A good quality pendulum is a must. Stainless steel is a good choice, and a wooden pendulum is okay too. I use a pendulum with a plastic body that has a good amount of weight to it. Crystal is not a good choice. You want as neutral a material as possible, heavy enough to swing easily.

Swing the pendulum in a back and forth motion to start. Become adept at getting "yes" and "no" answers to very simple questions:

"My name is Molly," or "My name is Lulubird." A clockwise swing indicates a "yes" answer while a counterclockwise swing indicates a "no" answer. (See illustration #3.)

Make your swings nice and big with a kind of free, loose energy. Beginners tend to hover over their pendulums making tight little swings, controlling everything with their left brain. This is not the best plan. You are working with your whole body here, not just the left brain. It took me a number of months of intense practice to feel "yes" or "no" answer in my whole body.

Be neutral when asking your questions. You are asking the body, not yourself. Staying neutral is harder than it looks! Everyone has an incredible number of beliefs lodged in their brain about how things work. For example, almost everyone believes that a certain amount of vitamin and mineral supplementation is necessary for the body every day. However, in asking the body you may get back an answer that contradicts this belief. I try to go with what the body says, not with what I think about it.

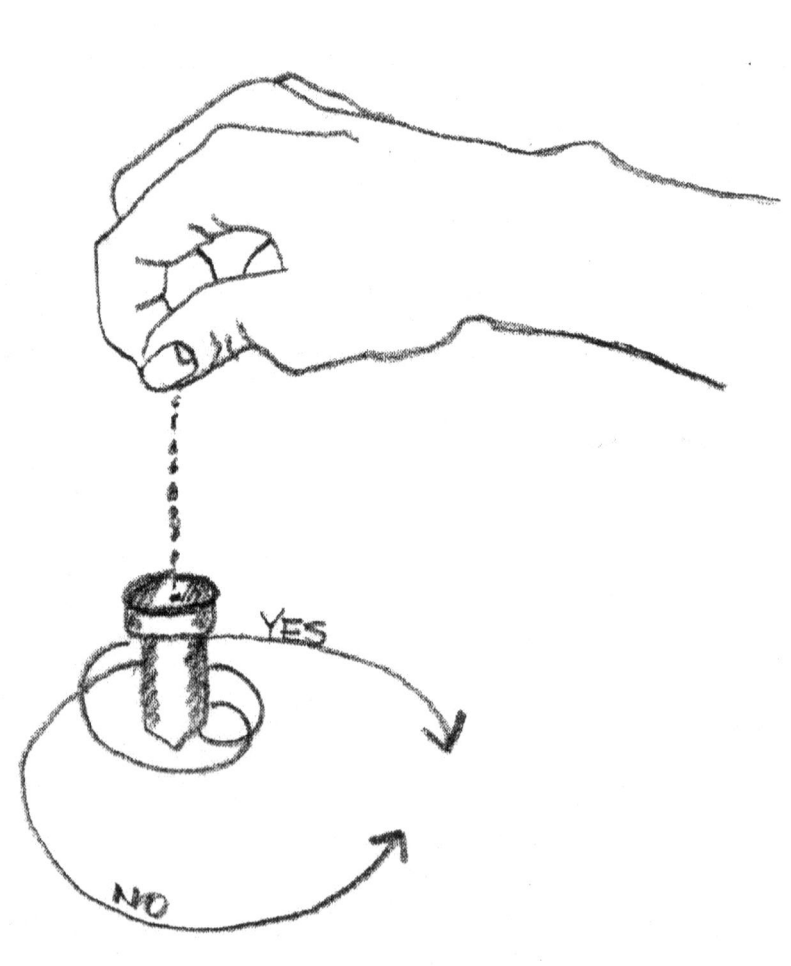

Below is a list of factors that can throw off your pendulum readings. These factors were determined by my taking hundreds of readings on many clients and double checking these readings with muscle testing. *Really* take these factors into account! Otherwise your readings will not be accurate and you will be off in la-la land somewhere. You will be getting "yes" and "no" answers from the body, but they will not be correct. You can *always* use the simpler technique of muscle testing if you need to.

1. Dehydration. The number one cause of inaccurate readings. I drink a lot of water when I am working, about a liter every 45 minutes. I drink every few minutes to make sure my readings are correct.

2. Leaning on the treatment table.

3. Client has crossed arms and/or legs. Client's legs are too far apart. The legs should be straight, not spread apart on the table.

4. Client is wearing too much synthetic clothing. (Bra and panties is okay, more may be a problem.)

5. You are wearing too much synthetic clothing.

6. You or the client has metal crossing the center line of the body - like jewelry or glasses with metal frames.

7. Battery powered watches *can* throw readings, but not usually.

8. You are too tired, your blood sugar is too low, you are way out of balance yourself.

9. Storms with lots of rain can throw my readings.

10. You have an agenda that you are imposing on the client. This is usually a belief about how things are supposed to work or a treatment protocol that you have difficulty relinquishing.

Molly Jones L.Ac., Dipl. Ac.

11. You are physically disconnected from the client and are not reading accurately because of this. I always put my hand on the client's arm so that I am connected to them while dowsing.

As with many techniques, the key to dowsing with a pendulum is *lots* of practice. You can always fall back on muscle testing to double check your readings when learning how to use a pendulum.

Chapter Four
How I Developed as an Intuitive Healer

Almost everybody has had psychic or intuitive experiences. Most people have answered the phone knowing who will be calling, for example. One time I was casually eating a handful of cashews. I suddenly looked down to find a piece of metal in the nuts, just before I was going to pop the last handful in my mouth. I "knew" something was wrong and I looked down in time to keep from eating the metal. Most people can testify to similar experiences. Although powerful psychic individuals are rare, such as the renowned healer Edgar Cayce, psychic or intuitive experiences are commonplace and not limited to a rare number of unusual individuals.

In recent years I have experienced a marked increase in my ability to read the patient's body through psychic or intuitive means. I have found this intuitive information to be largely accurate and reliable, and I use it all the time to treat people. The more I have trusted this information, the more I have been able to receive it and use it in my work.

What happened to me in recent years which has caused a marked increase in my psychic capacities? I believe it is from actual changes which have occurred in my brain and nervous system due to spiritual practice. I have been a devotee of Adi Da Samraj for over twenty years, and have had the opportunity to receive his Darshan, or spiritual transmission, many times. Adi Da Samraj transmits the power of the Divine directly to devotees in Darshan occasions. His purpose is to awaken devotees to God, or the truth.

When I have received Darshan I have felt a great love pour through Adi Da Samraj's body. At times I have seen white light emanating in waves from Adi Da Samraj's physical form. I have felt blissful and a deep sense of peace during and after these sittings. A sense of free or unbound consciousness also emanates from Adi Da Samraj.

In recent years I have been able to receive this spiritual transmission more fully. This has changed my body, especially my brain, and I have become more psychic as a result. (This result is a secondary effect, not the primary effect of realization of the divine reality.)

On one particular occasion of Darshan in 1997 I was able to sit very close to Adi Da Samraj. There were only about thirty other people there, and I was sitting about twenty feet away for an hour and a half. I felt a powerful, blissful, descending current emanating from Adi Da Samraj flowing through my body, starting from my head. If I tilted my head back slightly I felt as if a large stream of golden white nectar was flowing into my brain. It was like thick liquid light, vibrating at a very high level. I was in a very blissful, exalted state because of receiving Adi Da Samraj's Darshan.

Since that day my head has felt open at the top. My crown chakra (the center at the top of the head) is apparently open, and my ajna chakra (the third eye center) is more open than before. Although I felt my psychic capacities had increased a lot before that sitting, I have felt that there was a marked change in these capacities since then. Perhaps in the future these capabilities will increase further.

Over time I have become more sensitive to areas of the patient's body that are out of balance and need attention. I will find myself turning automatically to these areas because I know they are "off." I will also get a thought or visual impression that tells me what to do during a treatment. Sometimes it is a single impression, and sometimes it is a stream of intuited information about the patient and what needs to be done during the treatment.

Subtle visual impressions often appear before my eyes as I look at a patient's body. These impressions give me a feeling of what is out of balance in the patient and what needs to be worked on first. For example, one patient with chronic fatigue syndrome appeared to have a priority problem of inflamed nerve endings. I could see these inflamed areas all along her spinal cord in a subtle vision.

Sometimes the information I intuit is delightfully illogical. There is no theory in the world which could explain why doing that particular treatment would work to help this patient. However, if I carry out the treatment according to what I intuit, the results are most often successful.

My first acupuncture teacher was the late Professor J.R. Worsley, an exceptionally fine acupuncturist and healer. He treated me when I first arrived to study with him in 1976. I was in such bad shape he thought I would drop dead in the middle of his class. As this would have been an embarrassment for all concerned he decided to save my life instead. During the treatments he gave me I was able to witness firsthand what great healing capabilities he had.

Professor Worsley was the first person I ever met who could see subtle energy. On one occasion he needled some points on my back, removed them, then had me turn over. He stood and waited, watching. All at once I felt a subtle surge of energy move across the front of my body. He saw it happen, said "good," and the treatment was complete.

After Professor Worsley would treat me I would often have vivid dreams, or an emotional release. For example, one time he needled stomach 36, a point commonly used by many acupuncturists. However, when he did this point the results were remarkable. That night I had the most vivid dreams of plates of delicious food. In the morning I could hardly wait to run down and eat breakfast.

On another occasion he needled one point on my arm. My face turned beet red as waves of warmth moved through my body. I felt unusually open on an emotional level. Later, as I walked through a park on the way back to my hotel, I felt I could hear the language of trees as I walked by them. I felt this language was constantly available to anyone who would listen, if they were sensitive enough to it.

During a two year period in the 1980s I was blessed with the opportunity to work with a gifted clairvoyant healer, Thomas Hirsch, who also has the capability of seeing subtle energy. Thomas allowed me to hover around during many of his treatments of clients, and actually pointed out what he was seeing in terms of subtle energy patterns. I began to be able to see some of what he was showing me, and to trust that I could develop this capability more fully.

When a client lies on my treatment table, I always scan their body with my eyes. They always have their clothing on, but this doesn't affect my ability to read the subtle energetic patterns available through sight. The important thing in seeing subtle energy is to be relaxed and receptive. Staring at an area doesn't work very well, whereas quickly scanning with the eyes very slightly out of focus will reveal a lot of what is going on.

Some areas may have a random or confused vibration, indicating the energy is not moving properly. For example, the energy in the lower abdomen moves clockwise. If a person is not digesting their food properly, there may be a chaotic vibrational pattern visible just above the skin showing that the energy is not moving in a normal clockwise direction. Dark areas with decreased vibration indicate an area where energy is deficient or leaking. Scars often have this appearance.

I may also see subtle energy cords connected to the body, or breaks in the etheric body, which is the subtle energy body extending out from the physical body. I may intuit a condition in the body which I see visually. There may be abnormal crystals somewhere in the muscles, for example, or the visual impression of a tar like substance somewhere in the body.

I always work with my hands directly on the patient, often on their arm or torso as they are lying on the table. In this way I ensure I am receiving information that pertains directly to that patient. I also make sure I am grounded in practical ways. I wear flat comfortable shoes with orthotics (special supports) in them, make sure I am not tired, and I eat well and on time. I also make sure that neither myself or the patient is dehydrated, that neither one of us has our arms or legs crossed, and that I am not leaning on the treatment table. I have also found that touching synthetic materials can throw off my readings.

Many machines are available for reading various conditions of the body, and I pay close attention to the results of lab work as a way to pinpoint problems. Intuitive work should be done in conjunction with modern medical diagnosis.

Energetic diagnostic devices like the Voll and Bioset machines are very useful, but nowadays people trust machines more than they trust their own senses. If I had relied on diagnostic machines *too much* I probably would not have developed the ability to read the subtle energies of the body.

People may feel that the ability to read the subtle energetics of the body is only available to certain people. But actually everyone does this on some level all the time. People are constantly "reading" other people, environments, and animals on a subliminal level. A mother can instantly tell if her child is not feeling well by looking at them. However, in the case of intuitive healers this information is read consciously, and it may take years of reading in a therapeutic setting to develop these skills.

It is not necessary for a person to have these capabilities in order to be competent as a practitioner. But I have found that developing myself in this area has helped me become more effective as a healer.

Chapter Five
White Magic - Vibrational Medicine in Action, Revisited

Vibrational medicine includes such diverse modalities as homeopathy, radionics treatment, and vial based techniques. In this chapter I describe the vial based vibrational medicine techniques I have been drawn to study.

Any acupuncturist who is also trained in vial based vibrational medicine knows that this additional training gives you the ability to treat difficult problems at a deep level. Health problems resulting from chemical exposure, for example, can be treated much more effectively with vibrational medicine using acupuncture points than with standard acupuncture and herbs alone. It is acupuncture with a bullet.

The first vial based technique I studied was Nambudripad's Allergy Elimination Technique, developed by Dr. Devi Nambudripad. Dr. Devi developed this technique after struggling with her own severe food allergies for many years.

There is a standard protocol required for NAET practitioners to follow on *all* clients, which is to clear the ten basics. The basics include foods, vitamins and minerals. After the basics are cleared the practitioner may move on to clearing other vials based on hypothetical knowledge of various disease conditions. Clearing the basics may require more than ten treatments, as treatments may fail and require repeating. At the time I studied NAET there was also a 25 hour avoidance period of the substance after it was cleared.

I am indebted to Dr. Devi for opening up the world of vial based techniques to me, however, I am not an NAET practitioner. I use the NAET vials I have in the office, and may clear a vial using the standard NAET points for that purpose, but I do not follow the standard NAET protocol.

I live and practice on a small island in middle of the Pacific Ocean. When I would tell people that they would need at least ten treatments to clear their food allergies before I could do anything else for them I almost got laughed off the island. Perhaps this approach flies in a huge metropolitan area, but people on Kauai demand quicker results for less money.

It is not necessary to clear the NAET basics on everyone. What *is* necessary is *to treat each individual's priorities accurately*. Patients' health improves and vials clear automatically, including the basics, when you take this approach. Vials clear automatically because *it is all about energy*. If you perceive the vials as energetic symbols rather than the actual set-in-concrete *thing*, you are much better off.

I clear a food, vitamin, or mineral vial when it comes up as a priority. I also may clear a food, vitamin, or mineral if the client says they are having trouble eating it or taking it. In this case I always ask permission from the body before clearing the substance. I may need to do one or more priorities *before* clearing a particular substance so that the body is prepared for clearing it.

If the substance is the true priority or if the body gives permission to clear it, I rarely use an extended avoidance period as required by NAET protocol. When it is necessary to *repeatedly* clear vials it is a sure indicator that these vials are *not* the priority vials for a particular individual.

I have studied Jaffe-Mellor Technique and use their vials and vial clearing protocol when necessary. It is easy to menu the Jaffe-Mellor protocols and vials as their system is well organized and orderly. This makes finding a JMT priority easy.

One of my favorite techniques is Body Alignment Technique developed by Dr. Jeff Levin. BAT was developed by Dr. Levin after he suffered from severe health problems himself. It is a beautifully designed system of gentle balances done *based on individual priority*. The balances are so gentle they can be used on anyone who can't tolerate stronger treatment, including children, animals, and people afraid of acupuncture needles. The concept of treating the client's priority is the foundation of Body Alignment Technique. There are a few unusual vials included within this system. BAT is beautifully menued and I use the laminated BAT charts all the time.

In my practice I have merely expanded the concept of priority treatment to include *every detail of every technique I know* in the menu of what I offer each client. I also do not require myself to use one technique throughout a particular treatment. I may use acupuncture, clear a JMT vial with TBM protocol and then clear an NAET vial using an auricular acupuncture point, for example.

I have studied Total Body Modification, developed by the venerable Dr. Victor Frank. Dr. Frank also suffered from debilitating health problems and worked over many years to treat himself, his wife, and many others. His balances are more chiropractic like than other systems, including his vial clearing protocols. Thus, TBM balances are needle less and perfect for children and animals. I have found that it is possible to prioritize Module 1, thus drastically reducing the work necessary to clear this module.

Dr. Frank's vials are far, far superior to the vials made by computer offered through other systems. TBM vials are made in a different way using a radionics machine, and vibratory strength of the TBM vials is much greater than other vials. I can always feel this when I pick up the box of TBM vials. Thus, I use prefer to use TBM vials if at all possible.

I have included in the appendix section information about how to contact the NAET, BAT, JMT, and TBM organizations for practitioners who wish to study these techniques. The information in this book does not teach any of these modalities. I am teaching how to ask the body and work by priority, not divulging information about vibrational medicine techniques per se. Go to the source if you wish to study these techniques.

Every practitioner who wishes to work by priority should spend some time developing detailed menus of each modality they use so that priorities can be quickly determined. The lists I use are neat, orderly, and laminated with plastic so they are easy to use. Every system has an index or table of contents to organize the materials they offer. This information can be used to develop a detailed menu for each system.

Practitioners who wish to work within the standard protocols of NAET and TBM, for example, should certainly continue to do so. Once the standard protocols are complete you may then move on to working by priority based on asking the body.

Chapter Six
Treating Fatigue

Fatigue usually results from multiple factors that overlap. Each factor must be successfully treated in order for energy levels to improve and remain stable. And each person must be treated individually for specific causes, which can be varied and numerous. Common factors that affect many fatigued patients are discussed here. Unusual and/or illogical factors may also contribute to fatigue, and these can be discovered by asking the body.

Many people with fatigue have what appears to be latent or active viruses and/or bacteria in their system. These can be many or few, depending on the individual, and they can be cleared energetically. Viruses, bacteria, and other unknown factors can cause the patient to test weak energetically on their own blood. Thus, it may be necessary to clear a patient on their own blood, or their own blood in combination with other factors, in order to speed recovery. I have also cleared people on their own urine and/or hair when necessary.

Fatigued patients often have compromised digestion which needs careful, thorough treatment. Candida bloom is often present, and the acid/alkaline balance is frequently off. They may need to be treated for food allergies. These factors can be treated effectively as discussed in the next chapter.

Weakness on certain parasite vibrations may be apparent in the fatigued individual. This indicates the actual presence of parasites, and/or a susceptibility to infestation by parasites. When muscle testing parasite vials, any weakness found can be treated through the following two-part treatment protocol.

When treating for parasites, I determine the correct parasite vial to use, along with combination vials as necessary. If there are many parasite frequencies that the patient is weak on, it may not be necessary to strengthen on each one. By finding the priority parasite vibration, other parasite vials may be strengthened automatically. I usually prescribe an oral agent to help rid the body of parasites after the vibrational treatment. The correct oral agent, as well as the length of time to take it and the dosage, can be determined by asking the body.

I often use olive leaf extract as an effective oral agent following a vibrational parasite treatment. This supplement can also be used to help the body rid itself of bacteria, viruses, and yeast following vibrational treatments. Because it can bother people with weak digestion or cause die off reactions such as flu like symptoms, the dosage should be checked by asking the body and then double checked often. If an individual can't take olive leaf extract, I may use peppermint oil, black walnut hull, and/or wormwood tincture.

Many times patients tell me they have been on a parasite cleanse for weeks or even months. The common oral formulas they have taken include black walnut hull and wormwood. Often their digestion has suffered from the long-term use of these formulas. Other people may have used a frequency "zapper" to eliminate parasites. However, I have yet to find anyone who has used these techniques who tests strong on any parasite vials. In these cases I do not believe that the person has fully eliminated parasites or gained enough immunity to reinfestation by parasites. However, after treating with vibrational medicine I find that people are strong on specific parasite vibrations and that oral agents can give an extra boost to the vibrational treatment.

There may be thyroid function abnormalities in people with fatigue problems. Thyroid function can be determined by a blood test, especially checking TSH, and by taking deep armpit temperature readings for five days the first thing in the morning before arising. Readings should be 97.8 to 98.2 degrees Fahrenheit. Women should take their temperature starting the second day of menstruation because a temperature rise occurs around the time of ovulation, which can lead to an incorrect interpretation of the test.

There are balances in TBM and BAT aimed at normalizing thyroid function. It is also possible to approach this problem by strengthening vials pertaining to thyroid function and/or by taking kelp, which contains iodine. Obviously it is optimal to treat the thyroid in this way before prescribing any medication. However, often people are already on medication or do not wish to spend time trying to normalize thyroid function and wish to take medication.

M.D.'s usually prescribe synthyroid, which is T4 only. However, in testing people energetically I find that patients are weak on synthyroid. This weakness can be corrected with vibrational medicine so that their body can utilize it optimally.

Naturopaths may prescribe Armour thyroid, which is a glandular supplement made from cows containing T2, T3, and T4. It is not favored by M.D.'s because it does not deliver a consistent dosage. However, people usually test strong energetically to it. Whatever supplement or medication is taken, follow-up testing is needed to make sure it is working correctly.

One common cause of fatigue is anemia, which can be checked by a blood test. Women who have heavy menstrual cycles are often anemic, or on the borderline. Taking iron corrects the problem. However, iron supplements can cause constipation and digestive disturbances. I like to be sure the patient is strong energetically on the iron (minerals) vial so that their assimilation is maximized. The patient's condition relative to anemia should be verified by follow up lab work.

Emotional factors can cause fatigue because they cause depression. However, depression as a catch all diagnosis for fatigue is lazy medicine. If other factors for fatigue are being treated, emotional factors may need to be treated as well. In fact, one of the main strengths of vibrational medicine is the ability to treat emotional factors concurrent with physical treatment. The patient may need to take an antidepressant for a period of time, or may need emotional therapy. But merely putting someone on an antidepressant without investigating and treating other factors for fatigue is usually not productive.

Many people with fatigue, particularly chronic fatigue, have had deleterious chemical exposure which has weakened the energetic functioning of the body. This can include exposure to chemicals such as pesticides, herbicides, paint fumes, and recreational or prescription drugs. The energetic disturbances resulting from this exposure can be repaired with vibrational medicine. For example, in my own case I was routinely exposed to paint fumes as a child. My father was an artist, and I smelled paint fumes every day for years. It was necessary for me to be treated on the specific weaknesses to lacquer and lacquer thinner, paying particular attention to strengthening the brain and nervous system, until I was strong energetically on it.

Often people with fatigue have chronic subluxations of the spine which can be helped by chiropractic. In fact, chiropractic and vibrational medicine work very well together. Chiropractic deals primarily with the structural level, and vibrational medicine with the energetic level. Both techniques complement each other and work together to help many patients.

I read with interest other practitioners' ideas about the cause of fatigue, particularly chronic fatigue. Everything from undiagnosed encephalitis to a disruption of the Kreb's cycle has been cited as a probable cause. A chronically fatigued patient may be weak on hundreds of vials including parasites, bacteria, viruses (including Epstein Barr), immune system factors, foods, specific detailed factors in foods (such as individual sugars, amino acids, and trace minerals), environmental allergens, the encephalitis vial, chemicals, heavy metals, radiation, and so on.

While some factors, such as anemia or thyroid function, can be easily determined with lab work and treated immediately, the patient still shows a great many energetic weaknesses on vials. If the practitioner clears every weakness, one vial at a time, they will be treating the patient at their funeral. Although I do not have all the answers to this dilemma, I have found that treating by priority vial for each individual works beautifully to clear *many* problem vials, so they don't need to be cleared individually.

Now when I treat a patient. including fatigue patients with lots of problems, I always ask their body in detail what the priority treatment is and carry it out to the letter. Sometimes the priority treatment is a logical, straightforward matter, and sometimes it is illogical.

Finally, sometimes there are hidden factors in fatigue. You may find that a vial tests strong, but when you ask the body if there is a hidden problem, when challenging the body with the same vial, the arm gives a "yes" response. I use two designations to find hidden problem: one is "hidden", one is "very hidden". I use two hand signals to tell the body I am looking for hidden problems, although this is not necessary. A verbal question asking if there is a hidden or very hidden problem works just as well.

Sometimes you can "feel" a hidden problem when testing a vial. The reading is strong, but you can "feel" that there is a problem, and you will find it by probing with hidden questions and/or hand signals.

Hidden problems can occur with other conditions as well. I am always aware that there may be a hidden problem, particularly if I am having trouble getting a reading on a priority. If I can't get a reading for a priority I always ask if there is a hidden or very hidden problem before finishing the treatment. Case history #8 details work on a case with many hidden priorities.

Chapter Seven
Treating the Digestion

One of the first questions I ask a patient is, "How is your digestion?" because digestion plays such a key role in good health. Many people have digestive problems which affect them every day, such as gas and bloating, constipation, loose stools, undigested food in the stool, acid reflux (heartburn), and reactions to foods they are intolerant of. Some people have more severe conditions, such as chronic inflammation of the bowel and diverticulitis. Treating the digestion is often a key part of successful treatment, especially in people with chronic illness. In fact, it is safe to say that everyone with chronic illness has compromised digestion.

One of the keys to treating digestion is to reduce or eliminate the food intolerance that plagues people every day. (See case history #4.) This is a factor whether or not people are aware of specific foods that bother them. Fortunately, vibrational medicine works beautifully to eliminate food intolerance and normalize people's ability to digest and absorb foods. Each person is unique and the treatments are individualized accordingly

In treating someone with digestive disorders it is important to know exactly the organ or organs that are malfunctioning. Many people say something like, "My stomach is bothering me," while pointing to the region of their small intestine, or even the lower region of the large intestine. So when someone says their digestion is not up to par, I try to find out *exactly* what area they are talking about. By the end of the treatment I want the reading on that area to be normal.

Candida yeast occurs normally in the body. It is only when candida goes out of balance, or "blooms," that it becomes a problem. Any time someone comes in with digestive disturbances, I always suspect that candida may be part of the problem. Gas and bloating are the main digestive symptoms of candida. Women may have chronic yeast infections, and I have seen fungal yeast infections around the nails of both men and women, as well as chronically itching ears and a tendency to crave sweets and/or carbohydrates. (See case history #7.)

Although many other symptoms are supposedly connected with candida, I cannot vouch for that with any certainty. In my practice I have noticed that more women than men have an imbalance of candida, perhaps because most women have taken birth control pills at some point in their reproductive life. Antibiotics also encourage candida bloom because they throw the natural flora of the body out of balance, particularly with repeated or long-term use.

Whenever anyone has digestive complaints and tests weak on the candida mix vial (containing the vibratory frequencies of several strains of candida), I know that they will need work on this factor at some point during treatment.

Before I began to use vibrational medicine in my practice, I treated candida by advising people to follow a strict diet containing only protein (fish, chicken, meat, and tofu), non starchy vegetables such as salads (with lemon and oil dressing) and steamed vegetables like broccoli, and very small amounts of grain and unleavened bread. I also prescribed Chinese herbs, which worked to normalize candida in the system. This method worked fairly well, but people generally have trouble adhering to a strict diet for extended periods, and so it was a difficult protocol to follow.

Now I treat candida by having people follow the strict candida diet for a relatively short period of time. At the same time I strengthen people on the candida mix vial and any other adjunct vials as necessary, such as mold, yeast, and sugar. Finally, I often put them on an effective anti candida oral agent. Most often I use olive leaf extract or a high quality acidophilus, depending on what is best for the individual patient. This protocol is brief, and generally the patient will be through the process in three weeks or less.

The beauty of strengthening the patient on the vibratory frequency of candida is that this gives their body the chance to normalize candida within the system over the next few weeks. By following the candida diet during this short period of time the body has a chance to normalize itself, and the patient does not face a lengthy period on a strict diet. And the addition of either olive leaf extract or a high quality acidophilus gives the body an additional boost in getting rid of excessive candida.

Although the candida diet is as stated above, I always dowse people on exactly what the candida diet should be in their case. Some people can eat more grain than others, as well as some vinegar, and soy sauce or Bragg's Liquid Aminos, which are completely restricted for other people who have a worse case of candida. I also dowse to discover exactly how many days they should be on the diet, since that varies depending on the individual. Some people only have to be on the diet for a week, others as long as three weeks or longer. After this period of time is over, people will be able to eat a wider range of foods, although they should avoid concentrated sweets. alcohol, and white flour products.

In addition, I dowse as to what the best oral anti candida agent is for each person, so that each individual gets a substance that they are energetically strong on. I will check carefully to see which general systemic anti candida supplement (such as olive leaf extract and/or a high quality probio acidophilus) would be best for them, as well as which Chinese herbal formula is best for a local vaginal yeast problem in women. I also dowse each person on the best dosage for them individually, and the amount of time they will need to take it. Dowsed information like this is not necessarily 100 percent accurate, but it gives a good estimation of correct dosage and other factors.

Olive leaf extract in particular is a very strong anti fungal, anti viral and antibacterial compound. It is possible for a patient to experience "die off" reactions after taking olive leaf extract for several days, such as flu like symptoms, headaches, and fever. Die off reactions indicate that the substance is doing the job of killing yeast (and also bacteria and viruses if they are latent in the system.) People tend to want to quit taking olive leaf extract when this happens, so the best thing is to dowse their dosage accurately before giving it to them. If die off reactions still occur, they should reduce the dosage to a minimal amount (sometimes as little as half a capsule per day), and continue to take it.

Finally, since I am treating based on priority, in the case of candida it is possible to speed treatment by dowsing the adjunct vials based on priority as well. Often the practitioner can clear other adjunct factors by strengthening on the priority adjunct vial first. Sometimes the priority adjunct vial is illogical, but I have seen very good results in clearing an illogical adjunct vial with candida mix.

Unless someone is eating an all raw diet, or a diet that is nearly all raw, they may need to take enzymes. This is because the naturally occurring enzymes in food are easily destroyed by cooking, canning, and other forms of food processing. Thus, many people with digestive problems need enzyme support with each meal. They may also need hydrochloric acid for digestion of protein, again determined by asking the body.

Most people eat a diet heavy on grains and protein, and thus they will tend to be in a very acidic condition. This imbalance needs to be addressed in a great many patients, and is a particularly important factor in people with digestive problems. The body as a whole is slightly acidic - the average pH value of all body tissues is usually 6.6 to 6.8. (A reading above 7.0 is alkaline and below 7.0 is acidic.) The body tries to maintain a normal blood pH by getting rid of excess acids through the urine. Thus, the second morning's urine (before eating or drinking anything) can be checked with pH tape, which gives an accurate reading on how the body is dealing with what the patient ate the day before. Although there is some individual variation on a normal pH range, this second urine pH reading should be between 6.0 and 7.0, tending more toward 6.0.

The body can also be dowsed by muscle testing by asking simple "yes" or "no" questions on the general overall acid/alkaline balance in the body. This is the quickest way. It is surprisingly accurate, and I use it frequently.

Since most people eat a diet heavily reliant on acid forming foods, however, it is not common to find someone who is in an overly alkaline state. The best way to correct an overall acidic condition is to eat a diet consisting of more fruits and vegetables. Almost all fruits and vegetables, even citrus, are alkaline forming foods. (Although citrus seems to be acidic, its effect on the body is alkaline.) Beans are alkaline forming, and milk less so. All other foods are acid forming, including dairy products besides milk. Some nuts, such as peanuts and walnuts, are considered acid forming whereas others (including almonds) are relatively alkaline forming.

Some people are reluctant to change their diet, so they may need to take a supplement that is alkaline forming, such as AlkaGreen (made by Morton Systems). As long as the person tests strong energetically on it, they can take this supplement with good results.

Occasionally I see someone who has gone overboard on cleansing the colon by using enemas or colonics. Sometimes the person has fasted and is now having difficulty getting their digestion to work again, particularly the colon. I am generally in favor of purifying regimes such as fasting and colonics, provided they are applied judiciously to each individual patient as needed. Most people have never engaged in any purifying regime and are badly in need of the detoxifying effects it can provide. However, these regimes need to be applied very carefully so that people are in better shape afterwards, not worse shape.

In situations where someone has used colonics excessively, or has fasted and now cannot eat or cannot eliminate, often the colon reading is highly irregular. Great care needs to be taken to gently coax the system back to work. I try to find a substance that will aid their digestion, particularly the colon. It may be a Chinese herbal formula, psyllium, ground flax seeds, peppermint oil, or a similar substance.

Once I find something that brings the digestive system to a more normal reading (place the substance on the thymus and muscle test), I generally find that very small amounts will help the digestion. Also, people do well eating blended foods such as squash soup, or smoothies, which take very little work to digest. Acupuncture treatment during this time can also help, as well as BAT balances geared to the digestive system.

Most people benefit from taking lemon juice in water in the morning on an empty stomach, on a regular basis. This drink acts as a gentle detoxifying agent and stimulates the liver and gallbladder. Slight nausea after drinking lemon juice in the morning indicates that the system is toxic. Usually this nausea will pass after a few days of using lemon water to cleanse and stimulate the digestive system.

One of the simplest and best things people can do to help their digestion is to chew better. People typically chew a little and swallow chunks of food. Since there are no teeth anywhere in the digestive tract besides the mouth, these chunks go through just as they are when swallowed. It can take practice to reprogram yourself to chew each mouthful thoroughly, but it is worth the effort.

Chapter Eight
Treating Emotions

Emotions, thoughts, and beliefs (both positive and negative) have a strong energetic effect on people. If you silently project a positive thought about someone toward them, their body's energy will be strong. If you silently project a negative thought, they will often collapse energetically. This can be checked easily with muscle testing. Like actual substances, thoughts, beliefs, and emotions have specific vibrational patterns and can be strengthened energetically.

For example, my husband, Chuck, is the perfect guinea pig and a willing participant in my experiments. If I silently project the thought "You are a strong, sensitive, caring person," while muscle testing, his energy remains strong. If I silently project the thought, "You are lazy," his energy goes weak. His body picks up the vibrational pattern of the thoughts I am projecting toward him without my saying a word.

Most emotions, thoughts or beliefs that people have difficulty with cause the body to become weak energetically, even if they are not consciously aware of it. Through vibrational healing it is possible to strengthen the body so that these thoughts, beliefs, or emotions do not have this weakening effect. The person may still feel strongly about certain emotional situations or events, but they will have more capacity to deal with them without becoming flattened energetically.

For example, maybe a person endured an emotionally charged incident many years before. Every time they remember that incident they collapse energetically. Or perhaps a specific person causes them to collapse. People with chronic life problems in a certain area, for example earning money, will go weak when challenged energetically with beliefs about money. Using vibrational medicine it is possible to strengthen the patient on incidents, other people, beliefs, and emotions themselves. Sometimes these emotional issues are connected to a treatment on a particular substance such as a food, or they may be separate from any other substance being worked on.

A good example of a strictly emotional treatment happened when I treated Ben, a successful businessman. He didn't want to come in for treatment, since he was healthy and felt nothing was wrong with him. Yet his wife dragged him in and insisted he have treatment, thinking this would alleviate some emotional problems between them.

This put me in a bind. Here he was, lying on the treatment table, jovial, congenial, but basically unwilling to be treated. There was his wife in the waiting room, tapping her foot. Naturally when I went over him in the initial scan there was nothing wrong with him. He had no basic food intolerance either, he seemed healthy as a horse. Also, when I asked for permission to treat him by dowsing his body I got a definite "no." I was getting ready to send him home with no treatment when I decided to try one more thing.

At this point I rechecked all his organs on a "stress challenge," which is a technique I use to see how the organs act under stress. I simply state silently that I am now dowsing the body on a stress challenge and take new readings. Again, everything was perfect. Except the heart. On a challenge Ben's heart reading was very weak. I tapped his brain gently and silently communicated to him that the heart reading was weak, did I have permission to treat? The answer came back "yes."

The first treatment to energetically strengthen his heart was related to an emotional incident six years before. He was in the middle of a painful divorce, which had a strong effect on his young son. When he remembered a particular incident when his son was upset, the reading on his heart absolutely bottomed out. The information on this incident, including the time when it occurred and who was involved came directly as a result of my asking his body using muscle testing. When I told him the information I was getting, Ben remembered the exact incident and related it in full to me. I double-checked his body to make sure that this was the event he needed strengthening on, and it was.

The treatment itself was simple. As he remembered the incident I strengthened him energetically using the NAET emotional treatment protocol. The treatment took about fifteen minutes. At the end of that time his heart reading was strong and normal as he spoke about and remembered the incident. I went on to treat him several more times on an emotional level in relation to the divorce, and some other people and events.

It is possible to strengthen people on past incidents, as in Ben's case, as well as on beliefs, other people, and emotions themselves. You can muscle test someone as they are thinking of another person, for example, and see what their reaction is. If they collapse energetically it may be necessary to strengthen them on that person, particularly if it is someone they have a lot of contact with. Husbands can test weak on their wives and vice versa. Or an employee can test weak on their boss. This is obviously not an optimal situation!

The treatment is the same as when Ben was strengthened on the incident: While the person thinks of and feels the other person, they are strengthened energetically. There may be organs involved besides the heart, and these need to be strengthened as necessary. After the treatment the patient should test strong on the other person. They may not like them any better, but they will not be flattened energetically by their contact with them, and will usually be able to get along with them better as a result.

One married couple comes to mind whom I treated some time ago. The wife couldn't stand it when the husband collapsed and "played his victim number" (her words), especially when it came to his financial affairs. He couldn't stand it when she tried to take over, insisted on having her own way, and "tried to push him around" (his words). In testing other issues they weren't weak at all, only when I tested them on these particular ones. So I did two treatments, one on him and one on her. They imagined their partner engaged in the behavior they couldn't stand during the treatment, and afterwards they tested strong. During the weeks that followed they reported their relationship much improved. They weren't bugged by each other nearly as much, and the offending behaviors actually seemed to decrease.

People can be strengthened on beliefs as well. They may go totally weak when challenged by a belief, for example, "money flows right to me," or "spiders are good." In this case the patient merely has to hold the written belief in their hand during the treatment. They may also affirm the belief to themselves or aloud. Afterwards they will test strong on that belief.

Body Alignment Technique balances often have an emotional component, as mentioned in chapter two. Jeff Levin has formulated a long, comprehensive list of words associated with emotions, emotional states, and situations. When there is an emotional component in a BAT balance, this list can be scanned to find the appropriate emotion or emotions involved. This process is uncannily accurate. The words drawn from the list will invariably reflect the emotional core of an imbalance in the patient.

Treating people on an emotional level with vibrational medicine is quick and effective, and can be used in conjunction with other therapies if necessary. By using vibrational medicine, the patient may not need to have long courses of therapy where they repeatedly process incidents and events that occurred in the past.

Chapter Nine
Treating the Brain and Nervous System

Although there may be some exceptions that I am not familiar with, alternative medical techniques in general are not very effective in directly and specifically treating brain function. Chiropractic, homeopathy, acupuncture, and other alternative medical techniques may positively influence brain and nervous system function. However, I routinely find that people are still weak in these functional areas even with the use of these benign and positive techniques.

Although it might be the case that some people can *only* be helped with pharmacology, I have seen striking examples of clients being helped in the crucial area of brain function with vibrational medicine. I now check every patient for the energetic level of their brain function, using muscle testing or dowsing to scan all parts of the brain including the low or ancient brain in the area of the occiput, the temporal areas, and the frontal lobe. People with chronic illness invariably test abnormally in one or more of these areas. Many other people with less severe symptoms also test abnormally. People with abnormal brain function often show weakness on the bottoms of their feet as well.

In scanning or muscle testing I get an initial reading and also a deep reading, which checks the function in the deeper levels of the body, in this case, the brain. The deep reading is taken by mentally communicating to the patient's body that I am now dowsing for function at a deep level. Often this reading will be more abnormal than the initial (more superficial) reading. This technique can be done for other parts of the body as well.

In order to get the brain function reading to normalize, it is necessary for the practitioner to treat accurately by priority. I treat according to the patient's priority vial (or vials), which may or may not directly affect the brain, but I may strengthen the brain specifically as well. While they are being cleared on a vial, I will check brain function and make sure it is normalized by using specific acupuncture points. The Shenmen point in the ear usually works to accomplish this. There is also a special brain stem point in the ear that can be used if necessary. If these points do not strengthen brain function, the practitioner can ask the patient's body which point or points to use to accomplish this. Often a point such as Kidney 2 will work, or an illogical point (which makes no sense to the practitioner) will work beautifully. After using a point or points to strengthen brain function, I double-check by scanning the entire brain region by muscle testing, to make sure the brain function is strengthened.

With clients complaining of brain function problems (memory loss, depression and so on) I may also clear vials that are key to proper brain function, such as seratonin, dopamine, and chromium, again paying special attention to strengthening the brain itself during each treatment. I always ask permission before clearing any vial, and complete preparatory priorities if necessary before clearing a vial. All information on how to proceed is determined by asking the body.

Each time I clear a virus, bacteria, heavy metals, candida, and so on, I make sure the brain is strengthened as well, so that the whole body, including the brain, can normalize itself and rid itself of these negative substances and organisms. In working this way I have noticed that over time the brain function reading normalizes and becomes more stable.

BAT can be used with good results to strengthen brain function. Often the priority balance (or balances) will automatically lift brain function, and there are also balances that can be used involving specific points related directly to the brain to normalize brain function. One of the most common complaints associated with abnormal brain function is depression, and I have seen BAT balances work very well to bring up brain function and lift the accompanying depression.

Should the patient decide they want to take antidepressants, it is possible to normalize their response to the drug they are taking using vibrational medicine, thus minimizing side effects. Often patients respond to these drugs in a hyper mode, rather than a weakened response, but this abnormal reaction can also be normalized. In this case the body does not become weak when challenged by the substance when muscle tested. Rather the body reacts by becoming too strong and vibrating in a hyper functioning chaotic fashion. You may be able to see the hyper reaction visually when the body is challenged by a drug or a vial placed on the thymus.

I sometimes use a scale from 1 - 10 when testing a substance or a vial, to see how optimal a substance is for the body. If the substance produces a hyper reaction the arm will go weak somewhere higher than the upper value of 10: at 11, 12, 13, and so on. If a drug or vial produces a hyper reaction, simply ask the body how to correct this abnormal response and follow the instructions to the letter. Then the substance should muscle test within the normal range of 1 to 10.

People in modern society are routinely exposed to electromagnetic force fields from computers, cell phones, power lines, and so on. I have noticed that these can have a direct negative effect on the brain and nervous system. For example if you place the cell phone on the thymus, *everyone* goes weak when muscle tested.

Wearing a watch with a battery may make a person weak, particularly in the meridians or energy pathways on the arm that the watch is on. Working for hours on computers can have a negative energetic effect (except for laptops). With the exception of the guy sitting in the middle of the Amazon jungle, this problem is so serious, pervasive, and widespread that almost everyone would be helped by using vibrational medical techniques to counteract it.

These abnormal reactions can be strengthened with vibrational medicine treatment or by using specific energy tools (see below) which negate the effect of electromagnetic fields on the body. The practitioner can strengthen a patient while they are actually sitting in front of a computer or holding a cell phone, or they can use the radiation vial or electrostatic electricity vial. I have strengthened people on their cell phone while they are holding it, taking extra care to strengthen the brain and nervous system, as well as other systems as necessary. It may be necessary to use combination vials when clearing a cell phone or computer.

The BAT system has an electromagnetic balance that can be strengthened during a balance to normalize the body's reaction to electromagnetic force fields. Also available from BAT's developer, Jeff Levin, are vortex cards that work to normalize the body's reaction to electromagnetic equipment. These cards are encoded with an energetic vibration that normalizes the body's reaction to electromagnetic force fields, and they work beautifully. I purchased the square vortex card and taped it to my cell phone, solving the problem of my going weak when I picked it up. I have had it taped to my phone for several years and it still works fine.

Chapter Ten
Treating Bacterial and Viral Infections

Antibiotics are routinely over prescribed, often at the insistence of the patient. This has led to an ongoing worldwide crisis of antibiotic resistant strains of dangerous bacteria. The other morning as I was calmly reading the paper at breakfast, I saw an article about antibiotic resistant strains of tuberculosis originating in Russia and being spread around the world, primarily by people catching it on airplanes from infected passengers. After reading this I decided not to read the paper anymore while I am eating breakfast. However, this may not be a complete solution to the problem.

I have also read about antibiotic resistant strains of bubonic plague (spread by fleas which hitchhike on rats), as well as antibiotic resistant killer forms of bacterial infections that eat healthy tissue and cause death within a few hours. This is also not good breakfast reading.

Antibiotics, once deemed wonder drugs, seem to be losing the race with bacteria. A series of newer and stronger antibiotics have been developed, only to be eclipsed over time by stronger bacteria. These drugs are prescribed for common ailments, rather than being saved for truly necessary applications where the body is overwhelmed by infection and cannot be helped by more conservative means.

Antibiotics also have a negative effect on the immune system and wipe out the beneficial bacterial flora in the intestinal tract. While these bacteria can be replaced by using a good probiotic supplement, the long term negative effect on the immune system, particularly by repeated use of antibiotics, is more difficult to repair. I routinely see patients, primarily women, who were given both antibiotics and birth control pills over a long period of time, and have ended up with major chronic health concerns such as digestive problems from candida bloom, flagging energy, and the tendency to get sick often because of a weakened immune system.

People are understandably interested in herbal formulas for immune system enhancement. They come in with the flu or a bad cold wanting something that works well, and right away. While it is true that herbal formulas containing echinacea, golden seal, and garlic can help, often people are taking formulas that are not energetically optimal for them, thus mitigating their effectiveness.

In the appendix I have included a list of sources for effective immune system formulas including strong echinacea formulas, essential oils, and a source for Chinese patent herbal formulas for colds and flu. Echinacea should be taken in strong doses but only for short periods of time. Garlic formulas in dried powder form seem less potent than fresh garlic. I use fresh garlic water, made with three or four crushed cloves of garlic in a cup of water. After sitting for ten minutes, remove the garlic and drink the water for a potent anti viral, anti-bacterial drink.

Essential oils, especially peppermint and citrus blends, can be used over a long period of time to boost immunity. They can be sprayed into the air using a few drops in a cup of water in a spray bottle, or can be applied directly on the tongue in very small amounts. (I do this after I have seen a patient with a cold or flu.) Again, I *always check each substance on each patient* to be sure what is taken is energetically optimal for them, and to determine the correct dosage. If this is not done carefully the patient can react to what is given to them, or there will be no positive result from taking the substance.

When a client is already sick there are also bacteria/virus vials that can be strengthened using appropriate clearing protocols, depending on the individual. TBM in particular has very good protocols which work on various types of flu.

Sometimes these formulas and balances do not work, or work only partially, even if they muscle test as optimal for the patient. This is because the patient comes in already very sick and there are underlying chronic problems that have not been dealt with effectively. Coming in for a quick fix when you are already sick is a little like closing the barn door after the horse has run out.

People may have chronic, latent bacteria and/or viruses in their systems, and possibly candida problems, along with food allergies. They may have heavy metal toxicity due to having amalgam fillings in their teeth, or even after having their amalgams removed. All of these problems can be effectively dealt with using vibrational medicine. Again, I prefer to treat each person individually, working on the basis of their own priorities rather than on a standard set protocol, since each person will have unique findings.

The quality of the diet may need to be addressed. Again, this can be dowsed for each individual's unique circumstance. Infections can occur because the diet is toxifying the body, especially if the diet routinely includes substances such as sodas, hydrogenated fats, caffeinated drinks, and alcohol. Cigarettes, drugs and alcohol are especially toxifying. In these cases, how can the body fight infection effectively? I have seen remarkably quick results in resolving infections by putting a patient on a vegetable juice fast along with one or more cold water enemas to reduce fever and help the body dump toxins quickly. However, this does not always work, indicating that there are additional underlying factors affecting the body besides toxicity.

Once basic foundational work is completed clearing food intolerance, latent bacteria and/or viruses, candida problems, and so on, the immune system will invariably improve. The long term use of enzymes, a colloidal silver solution, and essential oils such as peppermint or citrus also boost the function of the immune system, as long as they are energetically optimal for the client. After people are treated in this fashion I have noticed that they get sick less often, and less severely.

The function of the sinuses is always compromised in people. In checking large numbers of patients I have yet to find someone with an initial normal reading on their sinuses. These findings corroborate the assertion of Kiiko Matsumoto, O.M.D., that no one who gets lung infections has healthy sinuses. She states that sinuses are the site of the first chronic infection in the body. Thus, working on improving the condition of the sinuses is of primary concern to improve the immune system and reduce the severity and frequency of infections.

In treating patients with vibrational medicine I make sure to strengthen the sinuses. Usually this happens automatically when accurately treating priorities. Occasionally that means using the sinus vial itself (as one of the adjunct vials). Sometimes it means bringing up the reading on the the sinus area by using specific acupuncture points determined in each individual's case by dowsing. For example, points affecting that part of the face may include those on the small intestine, colon, and/or stomach meridians.

People can make a big change in their sinuses by running a mild antibacterial solution up their nose so that it drains out of their mouth. Often there are pockets of infection where the nose empties into the back of the throat, and clearing these pockets helps the sinuses. With sinuses in bad condition this may need to be done several times on each nostril every day. A mild solution works well is salt water, at about the salinity of sea water. Irrigating the nose with salt water is an ancient yogic practice which, if done over a long enough period of time, markedly improves the condition of the sinuses.

My sinuses used to be in pretty bad condition, but I worked on them by snorting salt water several times for each nostril whenever I went swimming each week. Over time my sinuses have gotten a lot better, so I know this works. I have also seen many patients' sinuses improve by doing this practice over a period of time.

Chapter Eleven
Osteoporosis

Osteoporosis is the progressive thinning of bone in both men and women after the age of about 35. Men do not usually lose bone to the point of easy fractures, whereas women do. (The ratio of women to men is 5 to 1.) Approximately one quarter of all women will develop osteoporosis, so the threat is not great to a majority of women. However, for those who develop it, the complications of osteoporosis can be life threatening. An older woman with osteoporosis may break a hip in a fall, have difficulty healing, and develop further complications such as pneumonia, which can kill her. Bones in the spine can fracture and collapse causing dowager's hump, and bones in the wrist can also break and be difficult to heal.

There are several key risk factors for osteoporosis:

1. Women are more at risk, especially thin women and caucasian women.
2. Lack of physical exercise.
3. The ongoing use of certain medications such as corticosteriods (often given long-term to asthmatics), anticonvulsants, and heparin.
4. Diseases such as hyperthyroidism, hyperparathyroidism, kidney disease, liver disease, epilepsy, diabetes, and certain forms of cancer. Taking too much thyroid medication can cause

hyperthyroidism, having the same effect on the bones as the actual disease of hyperthyroidism.
5. Gum disease and tooth decay.
6. Cigarette smoking.
7. Consumption of caffeine and alcohol.
8. Early menopause or irregular menstrual cycles including, missed periods not caused by pregnancy and lactation.
9. A family history of osteoporosis on the maternal side.
10. Excess protein consumption.

The standard recommendations to combat osteoporosis include hormone replacement therapy (HRT), exercise, and an increased intake of calcium, primarily in the form of milk. Estrogen reduces the amount of calcium taken out of the bones, thus slowing osteoporosis. Studies have shown that taking estrogen replacement over long periods of time does reduce fractures, and also ameliorates other menopausal symptoms such as hot flashes, insomnia, and vaginal dryness. However, there are serious questions about the safety of long term HRT.

The body does whatever is necessary to balance calcium levels in the blood. There is a narrow range of optimal calcium blood levels, and dipping below these levels can be quickly life threatening, so the body will take calcium from bone if necessary to counteract an immediate threat. While HRT stops the body from taking calcium from the bone, no new bone is added with HRT. In addition, some studies show increased risk of breast and endometrial cancer from HRT, even with progesterone added as a buffer.

For example, in the Nurses Health Study released in 1995, which studied 122,000 women, there was a 36 percent increased chance of breast cancer when taking estrogen alone; a 50 percent increase when taking a combination of estrogen and progestin (a drug which has the essentially the same effects as progesterone); and a 78 percent increase when taking estrogen and testosterone together. In addition, researchers found that the longer a woman had taken estrogen and progesterone the greater the risk of breast cancer. This risk increased even more in older women (ages 60 to 64) who had been on HRT for five or more years. There have been other large studies since the Nurses Health Study which also showed very deleterious results when taking HRT.

There are three types of estrogen in the body...estrone (E1), estradiol (E2), and estriol (E3). All are made by the body in the ovary and the adrenal gland from cholesterol. Estrone makes estradiol, and vice versa. A negative effect of estradiol is that it can stimulate cell growth, in other words produce cancer, so there is a lifetime risk of exposure to estradiol. Estriol is produced by the ovaries by pregnant women, and is a safe type of estrogen because it does not have estradiol's cell growth effects. So women who have had one or more children reduce their life time exposure to estradiol during the months they are pregnant. In addition, there are now estrogen like substances in the environment (like plastics) which can take up estrogen sites in the cells and cause proliferation.

Estrogen compounds given now are "estrogen like" in their effect, and it is not fully known exactly how they will act in the body. Thus, the long-term effects of the use of HRT compounds are not completely understood at this time. Premarin, the most commonly prescribed HRT compound, is made from pregnant mare's urine, which is similar but not identical to human estrogen. It was thought that the addition of progesterone blocks the cell proliferation effect of estrogen. However, this does not appear to be the case. The long term effects of the use of progesterone or progestin substances alone are also not fully known. Studies have shown that progesterone slows bone loss, and may even stimulate bone building, but its effects on cell proliferation are not completely understood.

In addition, there are serious questions of animal abuse raised by groups such as the ASPCA concerning the methods used to harvest urine from pregnant mares who are restrained in their stalls. In addition, their young, unwanted foals are most often sold at auction for meat production. Frightened and confused at these auctions, they are often sold even before weaning age. Women would have second thoughts about taking Premarin if they directly saw the effect its production has on the mares and their foals.

Many doctors question the current trend to automatically prescribe HRT for menopausal women. For example, Susan Love, M.D., recommends in her book Dr. Susan Love's Hormone Book that before taking hormone replacement, a woman should consider her personal risk factors (listed earlier). A bone density test could be taken at about age 50. If bone density is low, she could make lifestyle changes, followed by a repeated bone density test in about five years, and every five years thereafter. Hormone replacement, if necessary, could start at about age 65. This reduces the amount of time a woman would be exposed to estrogen, since long term exposure increases risk.

Whether or not a woman decides to take standard hormone replacement, there are several very effective ways to counteract bone loss through diet, exercise, and elimination of certain habits such as smoking and alcohol and caffeine consumption.

Peak bone mass occurs by age 35, and is dependent on several factors (some genetic), early intake of calcium and vitamin D, and exercise. However, women of all ages can increase bone mass, even after fracturing a hip or other bones.

Calcium is a poorly absorbed mineral. Women dutifully take calcium pills, but they may not be dissolved, and they can go through the system essentially whole. A woman must have good digestive capacity, particularly from enzymes, in order to digest the calcium in pills. In addition, many women test weak energetically when muscle testing on calcium. This means they are not absorbing and utilizing calcium optimally. By strengthening them on the calcium mix vial using vibrational medicine, women will no longer be intolerant to several common forms of calcium, and will be able to absorb it better. Calcium is best taken with adequate water to avert the production of kidney stones.

Foods high in calcium include dairy products, nettles, collard greens, sesame seeds, and almonds. Nettle tea in particular is a very good source of usable calcium. Nettle tea made with fresh nettles dropped in simmering water tastes delicious. Nettles can also be ordered dried in bulk from any good herb company, such as Good Hope Botanicals. Too much fiber in the diet tends to stop adequate calcium production; however, that is not a concern for many people. Foods such as spinach, beets, and parsley containing oxalates tend to bind to calcium and hinder its absorption.

Interestingly enough, there are some tribal cultures with a very low calcium intake and low osteoporosis rates. Countries such as the U.S., U.K., and the Scandinavian countries have high osteoporosis rates by comparison. It is thought that high protein consumption in these countries contributes to the osteoporosis rate. If too much protein is consumed, the body will buffer the pH value of the blood with calcium, taking it from the bones if necessary.

The standard American and European diet typically includes several servings of animal protein a day, including eggs and perhaps ham, bacon, or sausage at breakfast; cheese, tuna, turkey, or other luncheon meats at lunch; and perhaps beef, chicken, or fish for dinner. Aside from the fact that this type of diet, high in animal protein, saturated fat, and low in fiber, has been shown in many studies to be deleterious to people's health, the addition of milk to a diet already high in protein merely adds to the protein load, the end result being the loss of calcium from the bones. Reducing the consumption of protein, particularly concentrated animal protein, is one of the keys to balancing the blood chemistry with regard to calcium.

Magnesium has been shown in studies to be just as important as calcium for building bone. Again, anyone with concerns about osteoporosis should be strengthened on magnesium if necessary, using vibrational medicine. There are good supplements containing both calcium and magnesium. I particularly recommend a calcium/ magnesium supplement (no. 16) made by Bronson Pharmaceutical Company. Bronson has a very good manufacturing process, and people are rarely intolerant to the fillers used in their supplements, whereas this is not the case with many of the other supplement companies that I have tested. Springreen Products sells a very fine liquid calcium/magnesium supplement called Calphonite, which can be ordered through a health professional. Liquid calcium is much easier to absorb than a pill, especially for older people with impaired digestion.

Again, each individual is unique and I prefer to test everyone on each supplement they are taking to make sure they are strong energetically on them. If they are not, I check other supplements to find the right one for them, or I spend a treatment session strengthening them on a supplement they are going to take. There is little benefit derived from taking foods and/or supplements that a person is intolerant to. This is where vibrational medicine shines as a practical technique used to reduce or eliminate intolerance to substances needed by the body.

Vitamin D and calcium are both necessary for actual bone production. Vitamin D combines with calcium in the kidneys to produce bone. Vitamin D is available when the body receives sunlight on the skin. It is also available in fortified cow's milk, but the drawbacks of relying heavily on dairy products has already been mentioned. To activate D only about 15 minutes of unscreened exposure to sunlight on a relatively small area like the arms or legs needs to be received. Short term exposure to sunlight to get adequate Vitamin D seems to outweigh other possible risks, such as skin cancer. I make it a point to get a few minutes of sunlight on my skin several times a week, without a sunscreen. I limit the amount of time I am exposed, and then put on sunscreen if I am going to stay out in the sun. I also do not shower immediately after being in the sun, as I understand it takes some time for the body to utilize the Vitamin D formed by the skin's exposure to sunlight.

Flaxseed is apparently anti carcinogenic, may prevent bone loss, and also contains omega 3 essential fatty acids. All of these factors are beneficial, so the addition of a small amount of ground flaxseed to the diet is optimal for women trying to ensure their long term health. There are naturally occurring estrogen inside pomegranate seeds and date seeds which may be used to boost estrogen levels, although no definitive studies on specific amounts to take have been done.

Besides diet, weight bearing exercise plays a key role in counteracting bone loss. By putting weight on the bones, the body is signaled to make more bone and lay it down in all bones of the body. Even women who have broken a bone can benefit from lifting small weights, as well as doing other weight bearing exercise such as walking with weights, and jogging. Bicycling uphill while putting a lot of downward pressure on the pedals has a weight bearing effect on the bones. Weight bearing exercise may be the key factor in staving off further bone loss in many women, including older women, and even Grandma can lift small three to five pound weights to signal her body to produce more bone.

Reducing alcohol and caffeine consumption and eliminating smoking have a marked effect on the body's ability to hold calcium in the bones. Drastically reducing or eliminating the consumption of carbonated drinks, including naturally carbonated waters, has a beneficial effect, since these beverages may adversely affect blood chemistry, causing calcium to be lost from the bones.

Some valuable Chinese herbal formulas can help treat the kidneys, in turn offsetting the effects of osteoporosis. In Oriental medical theory, the kidneys control the bones; these herbal formulas directly address that link. In particular I have used Osteoherbal, made by Health Concerns. Osteoherbal can be safely given unless there are symptoms of spleen deficiency (primarily indicated by digestive problems), in which case it is optimally used with another formula. Also, I make sure herbal formulas test strong energetically on the patient before giving them, since they may be allergic to them, in which case taking them would be counterproductive.

Menopausal symptoms such as hot flashes, mood swings, and vaginal dryness can often be treated successfully by using acupuncture, Chinese herbs, naturopathy and/or vibrational medicine. A competent practitioner in these modalities can help many women with menopausal symptoms, thus reducing the need to rely on a standard HRT prescription.

In Oriental medical theory jing essence *should* go down when a woman reaches menopausal age. The practice of artificially keeping hormone levels "normal" in current conventional and complementary medical systems puts an unnatural strain on certain meridian channels and organs in the body.

Thus, if a woman is experiencing menopausal symptoms it is best to go *first* to the most benign and least disruptive form of treatment including herbal formulas such as Two Immortals, Three Immortals, Abundant Yin and other related formulas. In addition, adequate good fats are needed in the diet such as flax seed oil, as well as B6, as these are dietary prerequisites for hormone production. (See case history #9.)

Many women will test weak energetically to the hormone vials estrogen, progesterone, or testosterone, indicating that their body is not utilizing their own hormones optimally. Using vibrational medicine it is possible to normalize the body's response and utilization of its own hormones with good results. BAT also has several hormonally related balances that work to normalize the body's hormonal balance.

If these least disruptive methods of treatment do not give enough symptomatic relief, the practitioner can then prescribe biologically equivalent or plant based estrogen and progesterone compounds such as those made by Beswecken. This class of compounds is probably safe, although no definitive long term studies have been done on them. Only as a last resort for symptomatic relief should conventional HRT be used.

Most prescription drugs test out weak energetically when patients are muscle tested, and patients complain of side effects because the body is not able to fully process these substances. I have found this to be true with HRT prescriptions, progesterone creams and pills, and birth control pills. Some prescription drugs cause the body to function in an energetically "hyper" mode. In either case, it is possible to correct the body's reaction to these substances so that the side effects are greatly reduced or eliminated. The results of this type of treatment can be seen immediately in the reduction or elimination of side effects; however, it is not yet known whether the long-term risks are reduced as well (such as the risk of cancer from HRT).

I have treated women successfully for unwanted side effects from birth control pills by using vibrational medicine. When clearing a prescription medication the practitioner asks the body *in detail* what protocol to use. There may be preparatory priorities necessary to complete before the actual medicine (with possible adjunct vials) is cleared.

Chapter Twelve
A Discussion of Diet

Diet is a rich and controversial subject. Everyone has an opinion about diet, feelings about the foods they like to eat, and memories of favorite childhood foods. Everyone has heard mainstream medical advice about diet, and read or heard about new books with new theories about the correct way to eat. In this chapter I discuss diet from the viewpoint of vibrational levels in different foods, and how the use of vibrational medicine can help to solve some of the problems people have with eating what will nourish them, as well as eating those foods that they enjoy. I start with the story of my own experimentation with diet and how my diet has evolved from what I ate during my earliest years.

My mother used to make lasagna with noodles, cottage cheese, regular cheese, and ground beef. She also made fish chowder with milk, fish, potatoes, and onions. And chicken and soft dumplings. She made apple pie with fresh apples, cinnamon, and homemade crust made with Crisco shortening. We drank lots of milk, ate Kraft singles cheese, Cheerios and Kix cereal, Wonder bread, and frozen vegetables. We ate desserts like chocolate cake, pie, and ice cream. We made delicious cinnamon toast with Wonder bread, sugar, cinnamon, and butter. We also threw Wonder bread (smashed into little balls) around the kitchen when she wasn't looking. She made Toll House cookies with lots of chocolate chips, butter, and sugar. We loved them, and so did all the neighborhood kids. She gave us liver (yuck) and always made a fresh salad out of iceberg lettuce.

One of my favorite dishes was tuna fish (out of a can), rice, and (frozen) peas.

I liked eating the food my mother made, but I don't eat that way anymore. My diet has changed slowly over time, through a lot of trial and error. I have experimented with many diets including vegan, less strict vegetarian, all raw, mostly raw, and very low carb diets.

I have fasted several times, including one supervised extended fast on water for seven days followed by three days on vegetable juice. The fast on water in particular seemed to clean and detoxify my system at a very deep cellular level. My daily diet is now moderate and simple, generally avoiding foods and drinks which toxify my system, such as refined carbohydrates, hydrogenated oils, soft drinks, caffeine, and alcohol.

Foods carry vibration, and some kinds of food have a higher vibratory frequency than others. Raw, fresh food has a higher vibratory frequency than cooked foods, for example. Rather than think of diet solely in terms of required food groups, I think of diet in terms of its vibrational quality, with the highest vibrational diets represented on one end of the scale by vegan and raw food regimes, and the lowest vibrational diets represented by diets consisting entirely (or almost entirely) of cooked foods, including killed foods, as well as other toxic substances including alcohol, caffeine, and sodas.

It is clear that eating a diet at the higher vibrational end of the scale is the next evolutionary step for people interested in spiritual practice. However, because I have a tendency toward hypoglycemia and metabolize food very quickly it is necessary for me to include animal protein in my diet. I try to get it from sources where animals are treated humanely, although this is not always possible.

There are strong cultural opinions against consuming a diet which contains a substantial amount of raw food. For example, in Chinese medical theory, raw food is to be avoided since it supposedly impairs digestion and causes the body to become cold. However, I have found as I have purified my system over the years that I want and need raw foods. I feel that the taboo in Chinese medicine against raw food exists in part because of a centuries old tradition of using human manure in agriculture in China. In this situation all foods must be cooked, since the risk of people getting parasites and infections from foods is so high otherwise. This risk is not the case in Western countries, however.

People can be cleared of their food intolerance using vibrational medicine, which is one of its strong points. People can also be cleared on weakness or intolerance to toxic substances such as coffee, alcohol, food additives, and so on. Sometimes these substances can't be avoided, or people do not want to avoid them. In these less than optimal cases it is possible to normalize the body's reaction to these substances so that the negative energetic effects are apparently reduced or eliminated.

Even extremely toxic substances such as pesticides and herbicides can be treated so that the body's reaction to them is apparently normalized. In this case the treatment appears to give the body the necessary means to rid itself of energetic toxic residues in the body, as well as an ongoing energetic capacity to deal with these substances as they are ingested. However, the long-term effects from this type of treatment, such as the possible reduction of cancer risk (given that these toxic substances have some role in causing cancer) have not been verified yet. Thus, it is optimal for people to maximize the amount of organically raised food in their diet.

Supplementation may still be necessary, but not to to the degree that many people are using it. I usually ask people to bring in everything they are currently taking so that I can check each supplement energetically on them. I check each supplement by placing it on the thymus and muscle testing. People usually bring in bags of supplements, sometimes 20 to 30 bottles! The amount they have spent on them is staggering! In checking them energetically, I find that they are usually weak (or hyper) on most if not all of them.

When you ask people if they like taking them, they usually say that they don't. They say that they force themselves to take them because they think they should, or that they forget to take them for days at a time. Both of these statements indicate that their bodies are rejecting these substances. People are acting on their mental theoretical knowledge, but meanwhile their bodies (no fools) are giving them the message not to take these substances because they are not energetically optimal for them. When this is the case the supplements weigh down the function of the body, throw it out of balance, and cause toxicity in the cells. If people really need to take a substance that is not energetically optimal for them, they can be treated to normalize their reaction to the substance using vibrational medicine.

Occasionally someone brings in a supplement or herbal formula that is energetically optimal for them. When you ask them if they like to take it, usually they are emphatic that they really do, a sign from their body that this particular substance is energetically optimal for them.

People generally don't need large quantities of supplements. Many people need a steady intake of enzymes and minerals, some probiotic supplementation, and possibly hydrochloric acid. They may need a good quality vitamin E, Vitamin A and/or a good quality B complex. All needs for supplementation can be determined for each individual by asking the body.

In doing a nutritional consultation I prefer to individually dowse each person's body on changes they need to make in terms of supplementation, their diet, and so on. I will generally go through a list of "yes" or "no" questions by dowsing to determine any changes the individual might need to make, such as: "Too much protein? Too little protein? Too much fat? Deficient in any vitamin? Deficient in Vitamin A? Deficient in Vitamin C? Deficient in any mineral?"… and so on. Once I find a problem area I determine exactly what change needs to be made, again by dowsing and asking "yes" or "no" questions.

For example, one woman came in needing to reduce her salt intake by 75 percent, a figure determined by dowsing. I was actually surprised by this figure until I asked her what she was eating, and she said she ate a lot of salt in the form of ham, chips, and so on. The figure apparently was accurate, determined by dowsing her body before I had asked her anything about her diet.

It is also possible to determine vitamin and mineral deficiencies with lab tests, and that can be done as well, particularly for people with severe chronic illnesses. These tests can be ordered by an M.D.,

N.D. or acupuncturist, depending on which state they are practicing in.

If a supplement is needed for a deficiency, such as B complex, I make sure that the one they take is energetically optimal for them before they take it. Even after determining they need to take B complex they may still test weak on a particular vitamin supplement containing B complex. This is because many supplements have fillers that people are intolerant of, or there are small amounts of toxic substances in the supplements left there from the manufacturing process. Apparently very few supplement companies have clean manufacturing processes, and people routinely test abnormally on many products.

Chinese herbal formulas are complex, often with many different herbal ingredients. Although they are formulated to fit many disease and imbalance conditions, I have found that often people are energetically intolerant to them. Thus, in using any herbal formula, including those using Chinese herbs and those using simpler Western herbs, I follow the same protocol, which involves muscle testing each individual before prescribing it. That means often I go through several formulas before finding one that works well for a particular individual.

Chapter Thirteen
Treating Addictions

People who are addicted to cigarettes, alcohol, recreational or prescription drugs test energetically either weak or hyper to them. Normalizing their body's response to these substances reduces or eliminates their craving, since craving a substance indicates an intolerance to it. Thus, vibrational medicine treatment may be the key to long term success for the addict.

For example, one patient with a history of alcohol abuse who had achieved periods of abstinence came in complaining that she was craving alcohol again and was having difficulty staying away from it. One treatment with NAET on alcohol reduced her craving, and she was then easily able to forego it.

Many people have taken or are taking recreational drugs including marijuana, hashish, LSD, peyote, heroin, cocaine, crystal meth, Quaaludes, Dexedrine and other forms of speed, and XTC. New forms of powerful drugs are developed every few years. For example, crack cocaine was developed after cocaine became a major drug of choice. It is more powerful, cheaper, and in wide use. Even marijuana has become much more potent over the years, now the potent resin containing flowers are used, resulting in a much stronger drug.

People like using drugs and alcohol. These substances lift people out of their normal bound patterns and give a sense of freedom. It is possible to use certain drugs in a sacred manner to explore the limits of consciousness. Peyote, for example, has been used in certain

Native American cultures in sacred ceremonies. However, usually drugs and alcohol are not used in sacred settings but in a random and chaotic fashion, often driven by gross addiction. Drugs and alcohol give a sense of freedom, but there is a physical price to pay.

In treating patients I will often find a priority treatment or series of treatments involving clearing a disturbance in the body caused by taking drugs and/or alcohol. Often this disturbance was laid down years before, but it lingers in the body's energetic pattern.

For example, one man in his forties who had not touched drugs since his college years almost thirty years before, had a series of priority treatments for LSD and cocaine. His body reacted with marked energetic weakness when challenged by the vials representing the vibrational frequencies of LSD and then cocaine. Another woman with severe health problems, including a very weak nervous system, had a series of priority treatments to clear crystal meth, cocaine, and marijuana.

Sugar is also a kind of a drug. People who crave sugar can be helped by using the TBM sugar protocols in particular. They may also need work on candida (plus adjunct vials like mold and alcohol) to eliminate sugar cravings. Often people need to reduce their total carbohydrate load, increase protein consumption, and drastically reduce refined carbohydrates in order to reduce sugar and carbohydrate cravings.

Chapter Fourteen
Treating Children and Animals

Children are fun to treat. Their imbalances are usually superficial and easy to correct. I have used both vibrational medicine on children with great results. With very young children I muscle test by using a surrogate, since young children don't understand how to resist when I muscle test them directly. The adult surrogate puts their hand on the child and then the muscle testing is done using the adult's other arm. The readings are thus the readings of the child, and you treat accordingly.

I have had beautiful results treating children with BAT. These treatments are completely painless, involving gently tapping and laying on of hands, and children like them. I have directly treated tiny infants with BAT with excellent results. TBM balances are also gentle, and thus good for children.

One such case involved a six week old baby named Allen. In reading his body I noticed a marked split between the upper and lower parts: above the waist was a normal reading, while below the waist was definitely deficient. He was crying and agitated, and his mother reported that he did not sleep well and was colicky. The first BAT treatment priority was a neurotransmitter balance. Three days later I saw him again, and a change was already apparent. His mother reported that he was sleeping better and much less colicky, and this time he lay peacefully on the treatment table during the treatment. He still had a slightly deficient reading, showing that more treatment was necessary. This time the priority treatment was a BAT hypothalamus balance. One final BAT treatment was done about two weeks later, and Allen has not had any more difficulty to date.

His mother wrote me this thank you note about two months after his last treatment: "I just wanted to take a minute and tell you how grateful I am for your help with Allen. I was skeptical at first, but the difference in Allen since your treatments is dramatic. He is happy, relaxed and colic free, day and night. Our entire family has benefited, less tension and a lot more smiles! Thank you so much!"

Animals can be treated with vibrational medicine with excellent results, again using a surrogate to muscle test. Animals are often plagued by allergies to the food and/or the water they are consuming, and can be treated for these problems. I have seen animals completely cured of severe (and visible) chronic parasitic infestations with NAET. I recommend animals be given optimal foods such as the Biologically Appropriate Raw Food patties. Animals can also be treated on an emotional level with vibrational medicine with good result.

Appendix 1
Resource List

Adi Da Samraj (information
about)

12040 N. Siegler Rd.
Middletown, Ca.
95461
(707) 928-4936
adidam.org

Ask the Body (This is Not
Rocket Science) Seminars
mailing list

Molly Jones L.Ac., Dipl. Ac.
115 Paako St.
Kapaa, Hi. 96746

Besweckan plant based
estrogen and progesterone

15495 SW Millikan Way
Beaverton, Oregon 97006
(503) 644-7800

Biologically Appropriate
Raw Food patties for animals

(866) 282-2273

Body Alignment Technique (BAT)	David Pasikov 3285 30th St. Suite 105 Boulder, Colorado 80301 (303) 442-6366 pasikov@email.com
Calcium/magnesium tablets #16	Bronson Pharmaceuticals (800) 525-8466 A company with a clean manufacturing process.
Calphonite…liquid calcium	Springreen Company (916) 347-5869
Cell Food…trace minerals, enzymes, amino acids	Dyna Pro (800) 877-1413
Chinese herbs: Osteoherbal	K'an Herbs (800) 543-5233
Chinese patent herbal formulas including patents for colds and flues and formulas for meno-pause	Mayway (800) 262-9929
Strong echinacea formulas	Dr. Schultz (888) 437-2362
Enzymes	Enzyme Formulations (800) 614-4400

Essential Oils	Young Living Essential Oils (800) 763-9963
Jaffe-Mellor Technique (JMT)	(866) 706-0712 jmt-jafmeltechnique.com
Korean hand magnets and acupuncture charts	Oriental Medical Supplies (800) 323-1839
Meridians of Chi Energy by J.R. Worsley	Redwing Reviews (800) 873-3946
Nambudripad's Allergy Elimination Technique (NAET)	6714 Beach Blvd. Buena Park, California 90621 (714) 523-8900
Nettles	Good Hope Botanicals (800) 577-7423
Olive Leaf Extract	PhytoPharmica (800) 553-2370
pH tape and Alka Green to balance pH	Morton Health Systems (800) 874-1478
Total Body Modification (TBM)	1140 E. Ft. Pierce Drive #27 St. George, Utah 84790 (435) 652-4340 tbmseminars.com

Strong herbal
patches and
formulas

Wei Labs
(888) 9191188

Appendix 2

Spend some time menuing for yourself - create detailed menus and laminate the finished products. This will make finding priorities faster and easier.

Sample Modalities Menu

acupuncture
allopathy
aryurveda
body work
chiropractic
colonics
counseling
cranio-sacral
dental work
detoxification
electromagnetic protection
exercise
herbs
homeopathy
massage
nutritional assessment

The modality menu can obviously be expanded to show a greater list of options. I use the expanded BAT modalities menu in my practice.

Sample Root Cause Menu

allergies
bacterial
candida
exhaustion
heavy metals
hormonal
infection
inflammation
malabsorbtion
mutated microorganisms
muscular/skeletal
nutrient deficiency
parasites
toxicity
vaccinations
viruses

The root cause menu can also be expanded to show a greater range of causes. I use the expanded BAT root cause menu in my practice.

Colors Menu

black
red
blue
violet
green
yellow
orange
white

Dietary Factors Menu

deficient/excess of:
Vitamin A
Vitamin B complex
    B1 (thiamin)
    B2 (riboflavin)
    B3 (niacin amine)
    B4
    B5 (pantothenic acid)
    B6
    B12
    B15
    folic acid
    biotin
    papa
    inositol
    choline
Vitamin C
Bioflavinoids
Anti-Oxidant factors
Essential Fatty Acids
    Omega 3
    Omega 6
Vitamin D
Vitamin E
Vitamin K
Protein
Carbohydrates
Acid/Alkaline factor
Minerals
    Trace minerals
    Calcium
    Potassium
    Magnesium
    Iron

Other menus you should optimally create for yourself:

Menu every detail of each separate modality you have studied.
Menu every vial you have in your office.
Menu every supplement, and herb you have in your office.
Menu every other tool you use for treatment in your office.
Menu every organ, gland, system and point for each part of the body.
Menu an emotions list - words that pertain to emotional states of all kinds.

Bibliography

Dean, Ward, M.D., and Charles, Jeff. *Anti Aging Bulletin*, Vol. 3, Issue 6 (August 1998).

Goldstein, Jay A., M.D. *Betrayal by the Brain*. New York: The Haworth Medical Press, 1996.

Gutzman, Holly, O.M.D. *Lectures on Prevention and Treatment of Osteoporosis*. Pacific Symposium, 1995.

John Hopkins Medical Handbook, New York: Rebus Inc., 1992.

Heritage, Ford. *Composition and Facts about Foods*. Health Research. California: Mekelumne, 1971

Kellosalmi, Ray, M.D. *"Hormones and Horses."* A.S.P.C.A. Animal Watch Magazine. Summer 1998.

Loomis, Howard F., D.C. *Enzyme Replacement Therapy*. Madison, Wisconsin: 21st Century Nutrition, 1996.

Loomis, Howard F., D.C. *Enzyme Replacement Therapy*. The American Chiropractor. 1997.

Love, Susan, M.D., and Lindsey, Karen. *Dr. Susan Love's Hormone Book*. New York: Random House,1997.

Matsumoto, Kiiko, O.M.D. *Lectures on Hara Diagnosis and Treatment of Sinus Disorders.* Pacific Symposium, 1989.

Nambudripad, Devi S., D.C. *Say Goodbye to Illness.* Buena Park, California: Delta Publishing Company, 1993.

Samraj, Adi Da. *Embrace my Discipline As Your Own: The "Minimum Optimum" Diet in the Way of the Heart.* Middletown, California: The Dawn Horse Press 1994.

Snyder, Arthur W., D.C. *Foods That Preserve the Alkaline Reserve.* Los Angeles: Hansen's, 1962.

Thomas, Helen, D.C. *Chronic Fatigue Syndrome.* 1st Annual NAET Symposium Booklet. Buena Park, California: Delta Publishing Company, 1995.

About the Author:

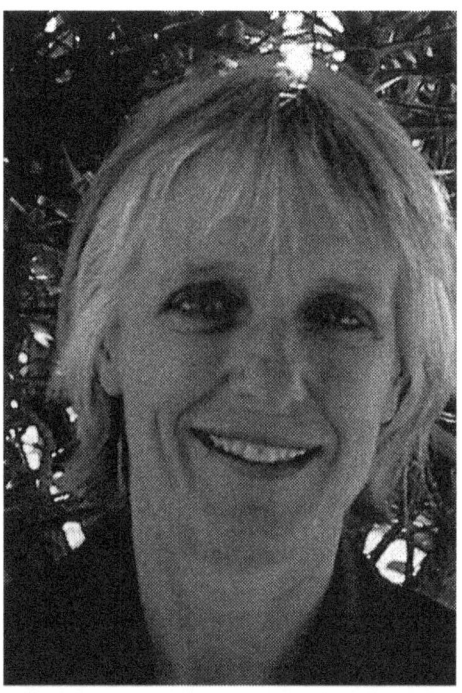

Molly Jones is a licensed acupuncturist (L.Ac.) in California (1979) and Hawaii (1989), NCAAOM certified as a Diplomat in Acupuncture. She graduated from The College of Traditional Chinese Acupuncture, U.K., in 1979, receiving Licentiate of Acupuncture and Bachelor of Acupuncture degrees. She currently has a private practice in Kapaa, Hawaii.

She is a graduate of beginning and advanced training in Nambudripad's Allergy Elimination Technique, Body Alignment Technique, Total Body Modification, and Jaffe-Mellor Technique. She has attended numerous other seminars and tutorials in Oriental Medicine and related topics, and appeared on the TV show *New Frontiers in Healing* where she was interviewed in depth about vibrational healing and preventing osteoporosis.

She lives in Hawaii with her husband and their golden retriever, and enjoys painting watercolors, swimming, biking, and snorkeling.

www.ingramcontent.com/pod-product-compliance
Lightning Source LLC
Chambersburg PA
CBHW030346290526
45785CB00004B/1622